THE
HEART DISEASE
COOKBOOK

Prevent and Reverse Heart Disease with 100 Heart Healthy Diet Recipes for Treatment & Reversal of Coronary Heart Disease, High Blood Pressure and Stroke Recovery

ELIZABETH HOLM

Printed in USA
ISBN-13: 978-1517752217
ISBN-10: 1517752213

CONTENTS

SALADS

LUNCH RECIPES

SOUP RECIPES

DINNER RECIPES

DESSERT RECIPES

YOU CAN EAT YOUR WAY OUT!

Guess what? There is a good chance that you've been misled for years or maybe even decades. For some time now, some doctors have been telling patients to watch their cholesterol. They claim that if it gets too high, persons may be at serious risk for heart disease or maybe even death. To make matters even worse, some doctors have been recommending prescription drugs to lower your cholesterol. Eventually, most of these drugs actually end up depleting the heart of certain essential nutrients that it needs to function optimally. Furthermore, some doctors have been guilty of ignoring the real reasons why so many people die from heart disease each year. Why would they ignore this? You may ask. I had asked myself the same question. Well, maybe it's just that they find it easier to just practice what they've been taught in medical school. Either way, it goes to show that doctors don't know everything. Interestingly, a renowned cardiac surgeon, Dr. Dwight Lundell, M.D. who had performed thousands of open heart surgeries and has seen into the hearts of over 5,000 patients has recently decided to change focus. Why? After his findings and such a wealth of experience, Dr. Lundell realized that something was missing from the puzzle. As a result, he decided to focus on the nutritional treatment of heart disease. Certainly, I agree. Focusing on good nutrition is the hallmark of preventing and reversing heart disease.

Now, many of us have been guilty of thinking that heart disease is a condition that affects older persons. But this really isn't so. When it comes to heart disease, age is just a number. Many cardiology superstars have seen serious cardiovascular pain and blockage among people in their 20s and also among people who are in their 90s. For this reason, many cardiologists have come to agree that heart disease can affect some people at almost any stage in life—even if they've been leading active lifestyles. Furthermore, according to Dr. Edward Palank, M.D., in recent years there has been an increase in the number of cardiovascular cases in young women and young smokers.

So, perhaps you or someone you know may be affected by coronary heart disease. Or, maybe you just simply want to avoid having to ever experience such a dreaded disease. Either way, you're reading the right book. The guidelines and recipes in this book will help you to easily prevent and reverse coronary heart disease; a killer disease in which sudden DEATH is the first symptom in over 60 percent of the cases. Now this is alarming! And no wonder, some people have dubbed it as "the silent killer", because, sometimes it really is. Now, maybe you're reading this and you've already had a heart attack, but luckily, you weren't a part of the grim statistics. Well, you should be thankful. You are now in a position to turn things around and live a happy and fulfilled life. Let's dig deeper.

UNDERSTANDING THE TYPES OF HEART DISEASE

There are many kinds of heart disease. Each condition may be caused by different circumstances and will have different and sometimes even similar symptoms. Many of the symptoms of the different types of heart disease may range from mild to severe depending on the condition. However, even if you are experiencing a few of these symptoms it may not necessarily mean that you are suffering from the particular disease. In case you have experienced any of these mentioned symptoms, please see your doctor for a thorough medical examination. Here are some common types of heart disease conditions and their symptoms:

- **Coronary Heart Disease:** According to statistics, Coronary Heart Disease, also known as CHD and commonly referred to as just "heart disease" is the number one killer in the United States, the United Kingdom and several other countries. It involves the narrowing or clogging of the coronary arteries that supply blood and oxygen to the heart. As a result, the area by the coronary artery is cut off from the blood supply, from the oxygen and from the nourishment carried by the blood. Eventually, the deprived area usually becomes severely damaged or destroyed. Symptoms may vary and may include: a mild discomfort in the middle of the chest area; feelings of mild indigestion; mild to severe pain beginning in the chest area and radiating up to the neck, face, back and down into the left arm; shortness of breath, blue lips or a state of shock.

- **Chest Pain**(Angina Pectoris): Angina pectoris, commonly called angina, refers to a squeezing chest pain that occurs when the heart isn't getting enough blood. When the plaque of atherosclerosis(cholesterol build-up) partially blocks an artery of the heart, the reduced blood flow can trigger an attack of angina. Typically, an attack of angina does not injure the heart if the heart muscle gets to quickly relax or rest. However, you should note that a person with an attack of angina is more likely to get a heart attack. Symptoms of angina may vary and may include: a mild discomfort in the middle of the chest area; feelings of mild indigestion; pain in the chest, neck or back. Bear in mind that not all chest pain or feelings of indigestion may be caused by angina.

- **Enlarged Heart** (Cardiomegaly): An enlarged heart is caused by undetected high blood pressure that had existed for a long period of time. Symptoms may vary and may include: shortness of breath, general low feelings, weakness and tiredness. Bear in mind that not all of these symptoms may be associated with cardiomegaly. Always check with your physician for further diagnosis.

- **Arrhythmia:** Arrhythmia describes any disorder in which the normal rhythm of the heart is disturbed. Whenever the heart's rhythm is increased by physical activity, it normally contracts in an orderly way. However, arrhythmia occurs when something goes wrong when the heart seeks to contract normally. Sometimes arrhythmia may not show any symptoms, however, some common symptoms are chest discomfort, palpitations, shortness of breath, dyspnoea, dizziness and anxiety.

- **Heart Valve Disease:** The heart has four valves which are responsible for ensuring that blood flows in the right direction. Heart valve disease occurs where there is a tightening of one or more of these valve which further results into what is called a heart murmur. It may also occur if a valve fails to open or close properly. While there may be no symptom at all, some emerging symptoms may include chest pain, fatigue, shortness of breath, light headedness, swelling of the legs and fainting.

- **Hypertrophic Cardiomyopathy:** Hypertrophic cardiomyopathy or HCM is believed to be a genetic disease and refers to an abnormal thickening of the walls of the heart which may result in a heart failure, diastolic dysfunction or even sudden death. Symptoms may include: shortness of breath, dizziness, heart failure and chest pain.

- **Pericarditis:** There is a little sac around the heart known as the pericardium. An infection of the pericardiumis called pericarditis which may result from inflammation or bacterial infection. Pericarditis has common symptoms such as a sharp chest pain in the middle of the chest, heart failure, swollen feet, fluid in the belly and shortness of breath.

- **Marfan Syndrome**: This is a genetic defect or disorder which results in the weakness of the connective tissues including those in the heart. Marfan syndrome can lead to progressive enlargement of the heart andit may further lead to sudden death in some cases. Marfan Syndrome may be undetected for a number of years, however, emerging symptoms may include: disproportionately long limbs, fin fingers and toes, indented or protruding chest bone, scoliosis, and near sightedness.

TAKING A DEEPER LOOK

As mentioned earlier, of all the diseases, coronary heart disease is still the number one killer in the United States and United Kingdom. Consequently, it is worth every effort to understand how to prevent and reverse such a lethal disease. Interestingly, if we should take a look at other countries we would realize that in some places, heart disease is almost nonexistent. In some parts of rural China and Africa for example, where their diet is almost entirely plant-based, heart disease rates are as low as 1%. On the other hand, in America and Britain, heart disease rates are soaring past 30%. Now, I find this quite heart breaking.

The good news is that coronary heart disease is about 90 percent (or more) preventable. In this book you'll learn how to prevent heart disease and even reverse it in some cases. Now, we couldn't look at curing heart disease without taking a quick look at obesity which is one of the leading risk factors for coronary heart disease. Based on data from the Center for Disease Control (CDC), since 1985, the rate of increase in obesity has become an epidemic in America. Today, there are over 9 million kids that are overweight in the U.S. alone. This further means that as these kids approach adulthood, they are also in the pipeline for developing coronary heart disease. Alarming isn't it? It's no wonder there are several speculations that over the next few decades or so, many parents may outlive their kids.

Well, many people have come to agree with those who theorize that obesity and heart disease is genetic. However, if we should analyze the statistics decades ago, we would realize that cases of heart disease and obesity were less prevalent. One major difference between then and now is that while our ancestors ate a lot of plant-based wholefoods then, today we are bombarded with processed and packaged foods. Most of the processed foods today contain a lot of fat, refined flour, salt and sugar. Processed meat for example usually has a significant portion of saturated fat, which happens to be the worst kind of fat that we could eat. The problem is that if we continue to eat a lot of fat, refined flour, salt and sugar, something is almost bound to go wrong. Ultimately, all these bad foods plus a few other factors will lead to the too main underlying causes of heart disease: inflammation and oxidative stress.

INFLAMMATION

Inflammation is a necessary process which happens in our body to help us to experience healing. However, if the inflammation process gets out of control, it can have devastating effects on the body. A study in 2002 revealed that instead of cholesterol, inflammation is the main cause of coronary heart disease. Further research has been done on C-reactive protein (CRP) levels and LDL cholesterol levels in over 20,000 menopausal women for about 8 years. They took keen notice of the women who ended up with cardiovascular problems and found that elevated levels of CRP was the best indicator of risk for cardiovascular issues. As a result, the researchers have formed the conclusion that the CRP level is a stronger indication of heart disease issues than LDL cholesterol levels. In other words, high inflammation poses a bigger problem with the risk of heart disease than high cholesterol.

OXIDATIVE STRESS

Oxidative stress interacts with cholesterol and this is what may have caused the cholesterol myth over the years. Now, cholesterol is not the bad guy that most doctors make it to be. In fact, it is a necessary raw material that is naturally made by the liver, brain and literally every cell in the body. Without cholesterol we would all die. Cholesterol is critical for the creation of hormones and cells as well as it is a major component of the surrounding cell membranes. This goes to show that cholesterol isn't such a bad thing after all. For decades, we have been cross-wired into believing that HDL is good cholesterol and that LDL is bad cholesterol. But, if we were to take either of these out of our body, it would literally collapse.

Let's look further. Our liver produces and regulates cholesterol, thus pushing cholesterol to the rest of our body. But the problem is, cholesterol is fat, while our blood is mostly water. And as we already know, fat doesn't mix well with water. Therefore, cholesterol

needs something like a "vehicle" to help it navigate through the blood stream to wherever it is needed. This is where HDL and LDL come in. In order to create this kind of vehicle, cholesterol is coated with a special protein and the resulting combined substance is called LDL (Low Density Lipoprotein). This LDL is then carried away into the bloodstream to wherever it is needed. As soon as the cells are finished processing the LDL, next HDL (High Density Lipoprotein) comes in like a garbage collector to scoop up any unused cholesterol. It then coats the unused cholesterol with another special protein in order to prepare it for transporting. The unused cholesterol is then carried back to the liver by HDL where it is then recycled or excreted from the body. By understanding the whole process we can come to realize that LDL and HDL are both critical components of our biology and neither is really "good" or "bad". Moreover, there is something that can happen to LDL which causes it to mutate into something that can really cause heart disease. Therefore, here is where we have a connection between inflammation, oxidative stress, cholesterol and heart disease. Additionally, LDL is just a mid-point in the entire process and should not be seen as the core factor for heart disease.

THE HEART ATTACK CONNECTION

Maybe you've already heard of the term "free radicals". Simply put, free radicals are unbalanced molecules that are missing an electron. Free radicals seek to rebalance themselves by stealing that missing electron from weaker molecules in the body. This in turn causes oxidization of those molecules and turns them into free radicals as well. As weird as these process sounds, it is actually a normal part of our biology which in turn involves breaking down the foods that we eat into energy. Now, our body has a built-in coping mechanism which rebalances free radicals using antioxidants that are either generated within the body or derived from mainly fruits and vegetables that we eat. By understanding this, we can further appreciate the importance of eating fresh fruits and vegetables. Biologically speaking, these antioxidants from wholefoods are very generous and carry around extra electrons which they kindly donate to the free radicals, thus causing them to rebalance.

However, it is important to understand that excess free radicals that are caused from a variety of poor lifestyle choices such as eating excess sugar or trans-fat, exposure to high stress levels, smoking or even a lack of exercise can override the body's ability to keep these free radicals in check. Ultimately, all this can lead to heart disease and a host of other chronic diseases. So, we can now conclude that one of the major causes of heart disease occurs when free radicals oxidize smaller LDL particles. After the arteries are damaged by these oxidized LDL particles, inflammation kicks in to help heal the damage caused. Inflammation does this by creating scarred tissue which is more commonly known as plaque. But the problem is that this same inflammation which is intended to heal starts to cause more damage to the arteries. A vicious cycle then ensues in which inflammation leads to more oxidative stress and vice versa. Consequently, more plaque begins to build up which results in further blockage of blood flow to the arteries. Furthermore, all this makes it more likely that blood clots will form in the arteries which could potentially lead to a heart attack.

3

EATING HEART SMART

From a dietary perspective, you need to know this. The ONLY diet that has been proven to prevent and reverse coronary heart disease in a large number of people is a plant-based diet. In fact, Cleveland Clinic researchers have recently confirmed that wholefoods can indeed cure heart disease. So, if a consistent plant-based diet can open up clogged arteries without drugs and without surgery and combat the number one killer, we need not look elsewhere. What we need to do is to seek out interesting ways to make plant-based foods a part of our daily diet. It's well worth the effort!

But let's be honest here, unless you're already a vegetarian, you may not really feel encouraged to eat mainly plant-based meals. Most people tend to think of fruits and vegetables as boring or bland foods. But in reality, fruits and vegetables are low on calories, high in antioxidants and other essential nutrients. And that's a winning combination right there. Therefore, if you really want to eat to support a healthy heart, then a plant-based lifestyle is definitely the way to go. For beginners, you are encouraged to try making the plant-based recipes in this book for 21 consecutive days. If you don't like it after 21 days, you can stop. Nevertheless, if you've decided to stick with it, then congratulations are in order. Your best days are ahead! Here is a quick-start eating guide below.

QUICK-START EATING GUIDE

Totally avoid oils. Oil may be useful for massages but we do not need to eat it. Most of us really use oil for sautéing, salad dressings and stir-fries, but we really don't need to use oil for this. Interestingly, almost any cooking liquid can be used to sauté or stir-fry vegetables, instead of oil. Here are some suggestions: purified water, no-sodium vegetable broth or stock and wine. Use cooking methods such as steaming, baking, and grilling, instead of frying. Oil-free baking may be a bit more challenging, however, useful oil substitutes include: no-sugar added apple butter and applesauce, pureed fruits such as apples, prunes and ripe bananas. There are also a few nut butter substitutes that you could consider (see the nuts section).

Totally avoid all animal proteins including meat, dairy, fish and eggs. Animal protein just simply isn't the best food for mankind. It is high in unhealthy fat, casein and cholesterol. Harvard research has shown that diets with animal protein have been found to increase the likelihood of coronary heart disease. While on the other hand, they have also found that diets that are high in plant protein had less risk factor for heart disease. Furthermore, other studies have shown that animal protein is high in l-carnitine, which is a non-essential amino acid that our body naturally manufactures by itself. When consumed, l-carnitine creates a certain gut flora profile. This gut flora in turn eats the food that we eat and gives off a by-product of l-carnitine known as TMAO (Trimethylamine N-oxide). TMOA has been implicated as one of the leading causes of arterial inflammation and ultimately leads to heart disease. Likewise, fish, meat and eggs also contribute to inflammation within the body. Therefore you should totally avoid all animal proteins and their "mock" vegan versions.

Use Himalayan salt in moderation. Maybe you've been told to avoid salt in the treatment of heart disease and high blood pressure. But, in this book you'll be told something different. Salt is an essential nutrient and contains sodium and chloride. A lack of sodium and chloride in the diet affects nerve impulses and normal cell functioning. In fact there are cells in our stomach which will not make stomach acids without salt. Further on, insufficient amounts of stomach acid lead to acid reflux due to an unhealthy stomach environment.

Generally, using any iodized salt with moderation should be fine. However, in this cookbook, Himalayan salt is recommended. Unlike regular iodized table salt which is synthesized in a lab and stripped of essential minerals, Himalayan salt is naturally mined from the earth. Furthermore, Himalayan salt naturally contains over 80 essential trace minerals that are needed for a healthy body and for boosting the cardiovascular system.

Totally avoid processed sugar and use natural sweeteners in moderation. All processed sugars such as brown sugar, white sugar, aspartame, splenda and others should be avoided. Instead, use the natural sweetness from sweet fruits such as mangos, grapes, bananas and no-sugar-added dried fruits (dates and raisins). You may also use a little honey or maple syrup when needed.

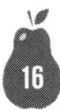

Eat lots of leafy greens, fruits and other vegetables. Leafy greens, fruits and vegetables are packed with essential nutrients such as vitamins, minerals and antioxidants. Healthy greens and vegetables that you should include in your daily diet are: broccoli, cauliflower, artichokes, arugula, asparagus, basil, beet greens, endive, bok choy, brussels sprouts, cabbage, celery, cilantro, collard greens, green onion, kale, lettuce, mustard, mushrooms, greens, parsley, rhubarb, salad greens, scallions, seaweed, spinach, Swiss chard, turnip greens, acorn squash, avocado, bell pepper, butternut squash cucumber, eggplant, green pepper, okra, olives, peppers, pumpkin, tomato, zucchini, beets, carrots, garlic, ginger, jicama, leeks, onions, potatoes radish, rutabaga, turnips and so on. Healthy fruits to include in your daily diet are: apples, bananas, blackberries, blueberries, cranberries, grapefruit, kiwi, lemon, mangoes, orange, papaya, pear, peach, raspberries, strawberries, watermelon, and so on.

Eat lots of legumes and whole grains. Legumes are full of nutrients and play an important role in the prevention of heart disease and other chronic diseases. Legumes should be a part of your daily diet and may significantly reduce the risk of high blood pressure and cardiovascular disease. Legumes are found to be great for maintaining healthy cholesterol levels. Healthy legumes to include in your daily diet are: adzuki beans, black beans, black-eyed peas, cannellini beans, chickpeas or garbanzo beans, green beans, kidney beans, lentils, lima beans, peas, pinto beans, soybeans or edamame, white beans and so on. Whole grains are also an essential part of a heart healthy diet and are well rated for their fibre-rich component. Examples of heart healthy wholegrains are: amaranth, barley, buckwheat, bulgur, corn, millet, oats (raw or old-fashioned), quinoa, rye, brown rice, sorghum, spelt, teff and wheat. Include whole grain by-products such as: oat flour, spelt flour, whole grain flour, whole wheat pastry flour, whole wheat couscous, brown rice pasta, whole grain pasta, whole wheat pasta, whole grain tortilla or sandwich wrap, whole wheat buns, whole wheat breadcrumbs, low-fat granola and so on.

Use spices and condiments. Sometimes you will want to spice things up a bit, even on a plant-based diet. Spices can be very useful in improving blood circulation and adding more flavour to your food. Here are some spices that you can use: basil, cilantro, dill, mint, oregano, parsley, rosemary, sage, tarragon, thyme, allspice, black pepper, caraway seeds, cayenne pepper, celery seeds, cinnamon, coriander, cumin, curry powder, garlic, ginger, nutmeg, onion, poppy seeds, pumpkin pie spice, paprika, smoked paprika and red pepper flakes. Also, you can use these condiments to add more flavour to your meals: non-fat low-sodium salsa, low-sodium hot sauce, low-sodium soy sauce, tomato sauce, no-sodium vegetable broth, vinegar (apple cider, balsamic, rice), wine, nutritional yeast, baking powder, baking soda, mint extract and vanilla extract.

Use some raw nuts. Not all nuts are good for the heart. For decades, there have been huge debates over whether or not nuts or nut butters should be allowed for a heart healthy diet at all. According to naturopath, Dr. James Rouse, a study was done on two groups of healthy Seventh Day Adventists with one group that ate little or no nuts and another group that ate nuts. This study revealed that, overtime, the group that had nuts had half the heart disease rates of the ones that had no nuts. So, this concludes that some nuts can play a positive role in heart health. Some nuts contain heart healthy nutrients such as monounsaturated fats, omega-3 fatty acids, folic acid and vitamin E. Now, this doesn't mean that you should get excited and overdo it, note that in everything moderation is the key. You should also note that peanuts and coconuts are not allowed. The heart healthy nuts are almonds, cashew, pistachio and walnuts. Raw nut butter and unsweetened nut milk from these heart healthy nuts can also be used in baking and otherwise. Do not use the processed oil from these nuts.

Drink lots of water. Water consumption isn't just recommended in the cure and prevention of heart disease, it is also essential for general good health. It is recommended that you drink up to 64 ounces of purified water daily.

SUBSTITUTION IDEAS

Even though this cookbook has a variety of recipes for everyone, for some reason or another you may want to make a few personal substitutions. Here are a few substitute suggestions:

- Substitute Avocado with Cooked Chayote Squash

- Substitute Almond Milk or Soy Milk with Organic Brown Rice Milk or Cashew Milk

- Substitute Nuts with Pumpkin Seeds

- Substitute Almond Butter with Organic Chia Seed Butter

POWERFUL FRIENDS OF THE HEART

GARLIC

In the world of fables, garlic is known to help ward off ghosts and vampires. But in the real world, studies have surfaced that have found that fresh garlic is helpful in warding off heart disease. A recent study by the University of Connecticut shows that raw crushed garlic generates a chemical which is known for its distinctive odour, hydrogen sulphide. The results showed that the consumption of raw garlic can help to relax the blood vessels and thus allowing an increased blood flow to pass through the heart. Furthermore, freshly crushed garlic has been shown to have powerful anti-inflammatory properties, antioxidant properties and also cholesterol lowering properties. However, you should note that cooked or processed garlic quickly loses its ability to generate hydrogen sulphide and therefore loses the heart health benefits. Therefore, if you do not have any restrictions due to certain pre-existing health conditions, then eating a clove of raw garlic daily is not a bad idea. Note that raw garlic is not usually recommended for persons suffering from low blood pressure.

GINGER

Ginger is a powerful natural spice which has been proven to reduce the risk of heart disease. It is a cheap and effective way to reduce oxidative stress and inflammation as you work on making better changes to your lifestyle. For decades, ginger has been used to treat conditions of the heart including high cholesterol and blood clots, thus reducing the risks of heart attack and stroke. Clinical studies have shown that ginger contains anti-inflammatory properties that work similarly to NSAIDs (nonsteroidal anti-inflammatory drugs). Even more specifically, ginger inhibits the action of several genes that are involved in the inflammation process and lowers cholesterol. The recommended amount of ginger extract is 5g per day or 2500mg twice per day. You can get more ginger into your diet by making ginger tea, taking organic ginger capsules or cooking with a little extra ginger. For making ginger tea, you may grate about an inch (2cm) of ginger and place it in a cup of freshly boiled water. Let the ginger seep in the water for about 3 minutes, then strain and enjoy.

SEVEN HEART NUGGETS

Here are seven (7) little nuggets that may help you to always have a healthy heart. Use these nuggets daily and you'll be amazed at the results:

1. Eat nutrient-dense organic plant-based foods

2. Moderate daily exercise

3. Minimize stress and negativism

4. Avoid toxic substances

5. Laugh out loud

6. Love and forgive

7. Be happy and grateful

JUST DO IT!

For years, many of us have been very successful in eating our way into heart disease. It is now time to eat our way out. By doing so, we may either end up reversing the damage that is already done or preventing any damage in the first place. With this cookbook, you

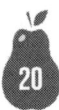

will be able to use organic wholefood recipes to nourish your system with super-nutrients that can save your heart. You should experience stunning results as you begin to eat more vegetables, fruits, beans and whole grains. You may notice that your cholesterol goes down, your weight goes down, your fat levels go down and then you will begin to experience a gradual melt-down of plaques in the arteries. That's great!

Now, if you have been eating animal-based foods, you may have to clear out your pantry. Go through some of the recipes and make a new shopping list. Read your labels and use the quick-start eating guide as a reference. Remember to always buy organic produce and remember to wash them properly before using. After you have prepared your pantry, your next step is to make the recipe. Follow the recipe directions carefully and enjoy your delicious wholesome meal. You can do this; your heart is counting on it. Just do it!

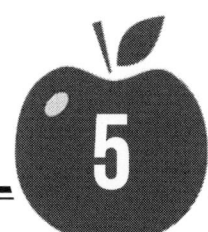

BREAKFAST RECIPES

TOFU & POTATO FRITTATA

This recipe makes an excellent frittata which is perfect for a breakfast. The tofu and potato combine very nicely in this recipe with the yeast.

MAKES: 4 servings
PREPARATION TIME: 15 minutes

COOKING TIME: 70 minutes

Ingredients

- ¼ cup sodium-free Vegetable Broth
- 1 White Onion, chopped
- 4 Scallions, chopped
- 3-4 Garlic Cloves, minced
- 2 medium Potatoes, peeled and sliced thinly
- 1 teaspoon Fresh Lemon juice

- Pinch of Red Pepper Flakes, crushed
- Freshly Ground Black Pepper, to taste
- 1¾ cups Silken Tofu, Extra Firm and pressed
- ¼ cup Nutritional Yeast
- ¼ cup Low-Sodium Soy Sauce

Directions

1. Preheat the oven to 350 degrees F and lightly grease a pie pan with sun butter.

2. In a skillet, heat 2 tablespoons of broth on a medium heat. Sauté the onion and scallions for 3 to 4 minutes before sautéing the garlic for about 1 minute. Add the remaining broth, potatoes, lemon juice, red pepper flakes and black pepper and cook, stirring occasionally, for 10 to 15 minutes. Transfer the potato mixture into the prepared pie pan.

3. Meanwhile, in a food processor add the remaining ingredients and pulse until well combined. Transfer the tofu mixture into the pie pan with the potato mixture and mix well. Bake for 45 to 50 minutes before removing from the oven. Let the dish cool for about 5 minutes before slicing.

OATMEAL & FRUIT BAKE

This recipe transforms the combination of oats and fruit into a classically delicious breakfast. The fresh fruits add a natural sweetness to this healthy bake whilst the oatmeal gives a lovely chewy topping.

MAKES: 4 servings

PREPARATION TIME: 15 minutes

COOKING TIME: 25 minutes

Ingredients

- ¾ cup Old-Fashioned Rolled Oats
- 2 tablespoons Unsweetened Applesauce
- ½ tablespoon Pure Maple Syrup
- 2 tablespoons Fresh Apple juice
- 2 tablespoons Whole Wheat Pastry Flour
- 1 teaspoon Ground Cinnamon
- 2 medium Peaches, peeled, pitted and chopped
- 2 cups Fresh Cherries, pitted and halved
- 1 teaspoon Corn Starch

Directions

1. Preheat the oven to 400 degrees F and lightly grease 4 ramekins with almond butter. Arrange the ramekins in a baking sheet.

2. In a bowl, mix together the oats, applesauce, maple syrup, 1 tablespoon of apple juice, flour and cinnamon. In another bowl, mix together the fruits, cornstarch and remaining apple juice. Transfer the mixture into the prepared ramekins and top with the oat mixture.

3. Bake for 20 to 25 minutes, or until the tops become golden brown.

BANANA & DATE BREAD

This super tasty bread is ideal for breakfast and kid's lunch boxes. The use of bananas and dates add moisture and natural sweetness to this bread.

MAKES: 4 servings
PREPARATION TIME: 15 minutes

COOKING TIME: 1 hour

Ingredients

- ⅓ cup Filtered Water
- 2 tablespoons Ground Flax Seeds
- 2 cups Whole Wheat Flour
- ½ teaspoon Baking Soda
- 1 teaspoon Baking Powder
- ½ teaspoon Ground Cinnamon
- Pinch of Himalayan Pink Salt

- 2 cups Ripe Banana, peeled and mashed
- ¼ cup Dates, pitted and chopped finely
- ¼ cup Almonds, chopped
- ½ teaspoons Vanilla Extract
- 2 tablespoons Sesame Seeds

Directions

1. Preheat the oven to 300 degrees F and line a loaf pan with parchment paper.

2. In a small bowl mix together the water and flax seeds, and set aside for 5 to 10 minutes. In a large bowl combine together the baking soda, baking powder, flour, cinnamon and salt. Fold in the banana, dates, almonds and vanilla. Combine the flax seed mixture with the flour mixture and knead until a dough forms. Transfer the dough into the prepared loaf pan. Top with sesame seeds.

3. Bake for 50 to 60 minutes, or until a toothpick inserted into the center comes out clean.

HEARTY FRENCH TOAST

These French toasts are very moist with a slight crispy touch. The use of mashed banana adds a wonderful sweetness to this toast. These toasts are a great hit for slow weekend breakfasts, and are a quick and easy breakfast.

MAKES: 2 servings

PREPARATION TIME: 15 minutes

COOKING TIME: 8 minutes

Ingredients

- 1¼ cups Almond Milk
- ½ cup Banana, peeled and mashed
- ½ tablespoon Flax Seeds
- 1 tablespoon Almond Meal
- ½ teaspoon Vanilla Extract
- ¼ teaspoon Ground Cinnamon
- 4 Whole Wheat Bread Slices

Directions

1. In a large bowl mix together all of the ingredients, except for the bread slices and almond meal. Set aside for at least 5 minutes.

2. Heat a large nonstick skillet on a medium heat. Dip a slice of bread into the banana mixture and coat evenly. Carefully place the bread into the skillet and sprinkle with a small amount of the almond meal. Cook for 3 to 4 minutes on each side. Repeat for the remaining bread slices.

VEGETABLE OMELETTE

This omelette, made with chickpea flour, has a delicious crunch of vegetables. With a side of salad this omelette is perfect for a satisfying breakfast. This omelette also makes a great addition to a kid's school lunch box.

MAKES: 2 servings

COOKING TIME: 20 minutes

PREPARATION TIME: 15 minutes

Ingredients

- 1 cup Warm Water
- 2 tablespoons Flax Meal
- 2 tablespoons Chia Seeds Meal
- Pinch of Red Pepper Flakes, crushed
- ⅛ teaspoon Himalayan Pink Salt
- ¾ cup Chickpea Flour
- 1 teaspoon Baking Powder
- 2 teaspoons Nutritional Yeast

- ¼ cup Green Bell Pepper, seeded and chopped
- ¼ cup Baby Bella Mushrooms, chopped
- ¼ cup Onion, chopped
- ½ cup Fresh Kale, trimmed and chopped
- 1 Serrano Chile, seeded and chopped
- 2 teaspoons Almond Butter

Directions

1. In a large bowl, mix together ½ cup of water and the flax meal. Set aside for about 5 minutes before stirring in the remaining water, chia seeds and seasoning. In another bowl, mix together the chickpea flour and baking powder before mixing the chickpea flour into the flax meal mixture. Fold in the nutritional yeast and vegetables.

2. Grease a large nonstick frying pan with 1 teaspoon of Almond butter and heat on a medium heat. Add the vegetable mixture and spread evenly in the frying pan. Cover and cook for about 6 to 7 minutes. Uncover the pan and pour in the remaining butter. Cook for a further 6 to 7 minutes. Carefully flip the omelette and cook for 5 to 6 minutes more.

SWEET POTATO PANCAKES

This recipe provides a wonderful change from regular pancakes, and it will create an impressive and fabulous breakfast, ideal for weekends. These pancakes are not only delicious, but super healthy too. Enjoy these pancakes with a topping of desired fresh berries.

MAKES: 4 servings

COOKING TIME: 5 minutes

PREPARATION TIME: 10 minutes (plus time to rest)

Ingredients

- ½ cup Spelt Flour
- ½ cup Whole Wheat Pastry Flour
- 1 tablespoon Ground Flax Seeds
- 2 teaspoons Baking Powder
- ½ teaspoon Ground Cinnamon
- ¼ teaspoon Ground Ginger
- ¼ teaspoon Ground Nutmeg
- Pinch of Ground Cloves
- 1 cup Unsweetened Almond Milk
- ⅓ cup Sweet Potato Puree
- ½ tablespoon Pure Maple Syrup
- ½ teaspoon Pure Vanilla Extract
- 1 tablespoon Almond Butter

Directions

1. In a bowl, mix together the flours, flax seeds, baking powder and spices. In another bowl, beat together the remaining ingredients, except for the almond butter. Mix the almond milk mixture into the flour mixture and set aside for 10 minutes.

2. Preheat the nonstick griddle on a medium-high heat and lightly grease with the almond butter. Pour ⅓ cup of the mixture into the griddle and, with a ladle, flatten slightly. Cook for 2 to 3 minutes before turning and cooking for 1 to 2 minutes more. Repeat with the remaining mixture.

SPICED PUMPKIN SMOOTHIE

This is one of the best and most delicious smoothies with a fantastic creamy texture. This smoothie will be a wonderful addition to your breakfast menu in the fall season.

MAKES: 2 servings　　　　　　　　**PREPARATION TIME:** 10 minutes

Ingredients

- ¾ cup Pumpkin Puree
- 3-4 Medjool Dates
- 1½ cups unsweetened Soy or Almond Milk
- 1 teaspoon Vanilla Extract
- 1 tablespoon Ground Chia Seeds

- ½ teaspoon Ground Ginger
- 1 teaspoon Ground Cinnamon
- Pinch of Ground Cloves
- ¼ cup Ice Cubes

Directions

1. In a blender, add all of the ingredients and pulse until smooth.

2. Pour the smoothie into glasses and serve immediately.

SEED & HERB FLAT BREAD

This is a quick and easily prepared healthy breakfast bread which has amazing flavors. This recipe makes a power packed seed bread which is really hearty, dense and tasty. It will be a great hit if served with almond butter.

MAKES: 4 servings   **COOKING TIME:** 25 minutes

PREPARATION TIME: 10 minutes

Ingredients

- ¼ cup Buckwheat Flour
- ½ cup Oat Flour
- ½ cup Pumpkin Seeds
- ½ cup Sunflower Seeds
- ½ cup Chia Seeds
- 1 teaspoon Fresh Thyme, minced

- 1 teaspoon Fresh Rosemary, minced
- ⅛ teaspoon Himalayan Pink Salt
- ½ teaspoon Pure Maple Syrup
- 1 cup Filtered Water
- ¼ cup Walnuts, toasted and chopped

Directions

1. Preheat the oven to 325 degrees F and line a 9-inch sized square baking pan with parchment paper.

2. In a large bowl, mix together all of the ingredients, except for the water and walnuts. Slowly add the water and mix until well combined before folding in the walnuts. Transfer the mixture into the prepared baking pan and bake for about 25 minutes.

VANILLA WAFFLES

This recipe is a special breakfast recipe for a lazy and rushed weekday morning. It is a great way to add healthy elements into your breakfast in a delicious way. These waffles have a nice and dense texture and a topping of almond butter will provide extra taste when serving.

MAKES: 2 servings

COOKING TIME: 5 minutes

PREPARATION TIME: 10 minutes

Ingredients

- ½ cup Spelt Flour
- 1 teaspoon Baking Powder
- ½ teaspoon Baking Soda
- Pinch of Himalayan Pink Salt
- 1 tablespoon unsweetened Almond Milk

- ½ cup Unsweetened Applesauce
- 2 tablespoons Pure Maple Syrup
- 1½ teaspoons Vanilla Extract
- 1 tablespoon Almond Butter

Directions

1. Add the flour, salt, baking powder and baking soda to a small bowl and mix together. In another bowl, beat together all of the remaining ingredients, except for the almond butter. Mix the almond milk mixture into the flour mixture.

2. Preheat the waffle iron according to the manufacturer's directions and grease the waffle iron with the almond butter. Add ½ of the mixture and cook for 4 to 5 minutes before repeating with the remaining mixture.

SPICED QUINOA BLUEBERRIES

This is a healthy and protein rich breakfast recipe that is quick and easy to prepare. Sweet ripe blackberries and crunchy walnuts compliments nicely with the chewy texture of the spiced quinoa.

MAKES: 4 servings

COOKING TIME: 20 minutes

PREPARATION TIME: 10 minutes

Ingredients

- 1 cup unsweetened Almond Milk
- 1 cup Filtered Water
- 1 cup Uncooked Quinoa, rinsed and strained
- 1 teaspoon Ground Cinnamon
- ¼ teaspoon Ground Ginger
- Pinch of Ground Nutmeg
- Pinch of Ground Cloves
- 2 tablespoons Pure Maple Syrup
- 2 cups Fresh Blueberries
- ¼ cup Walnuts, toasted and chopped

Directions

1. In a large pan, add the almond milk, water, quinoa and spices and bring to a boil on a medium heat. Cook for about 5 minutes before reducing the heat to medium-low. Simmer for about 15 minutes, uncovered, before removing the pan from the heat and setting aside, covered, for about 5 minutes.

2. Stir in the maple syrup and transfer into serving bowls. Top with blueberries and walnuts and serve.

FRUITY BAKED QUINOA

This recipe makes a healthy and delicious quinoa dish for weekend breakfasts. It provides healthy nutrition and works well for those picky eaters in the family!

MAKES: 4 servings

COOKING TIME: 50 minutes

PREPARATION TIME: 10 minutes

Ingredients

- 2½ cups unsweetened Almond Milk
- 1 cup Quinoa, rinsed and drained
- 1½ cups Pears, peeled, cored and chopped
- 2 Dates, pitted and chopped
- ¼ cup Golden Raisins
- ½ tablespoon Almond Butter
- 1½ teaspoons Ground Cinnamon
- Pinch of Ground Cloves
- Pinch of Ground Nutmeg

Directions

1. Preheat the oven to 375 degrees F and arrange the oven rack in the centre of the oven.

2. Mix together all of the ingredients in a large casserole dish. Tightly cover the dish with a large piece of foil paper and bake until cooked, for 45 to 50 minutes.

PUMPKIN BREAD CASSEROLE

This is a creative and a delicious way to use day-old bread for breakfast. This bread casserole is packed with the flavors of pumpkin and warm spices. Grilling this dish provides a crusty topping to this casserole.

MAKES: 2 servings

PREPARATION TIME: 15 minutes

COOKING TIME: 33 minutes

Ingredients

- ⅓ cup Filtered Water
- 2 tablespoons Ground Flax Seeds
- 2 tablespoons Almond Milk
- 2 tablespoons Pumpkin Puree
- ½ tablespoon Pure Maple Syrup
- ½ teaspoon Ground Cinnamon
- ¼ teaspoon Ground Ginger
- Pinch of Allspice
- Pinch of Ground Nutmeg
- Pinch of Ground Cloves
- Pinch of Himalayan Pink Salt
- ½ teaspoon Pure Vanilla Extract
- 3 cups day-old cubed Whole Wheat Bread Slices
- 1 Banana, peeled and sliced
- 2 tablespoons Walnuts, chopped

Directions

1. Preheat the oven to 350 degrees F and line a small baking dish with parchment paper. Generously grease a piece of foil paper with almond butter and set aside.

2. In a large bowl, mix together the water and flax seeds and set aside for 5 to 10 minutes. Add the milk, pumpkin puree, maple syrup and spices and beat until well combined. Carefully stir in the bread cubes until they are coated. Transfer the mixture into a prepared baking pan and cover with the prepared foil paper. Bake for about 25 minutes before removing the foil paper and baking for a further 5 minutes.

3. Remove the dish from the oven. Evenly place the banana slices and walnuts on top before grilling the dish for 2 to 3 minutes before serving.

FRUIT & NUT PORRIDGE

This delicious porridge is a healthy way to start your day. It is one of the most satisfying, nutritious and delicious recipes for breakfast. The use of almond milk in this dish adds a special creamy texture, and the mashed bananas gives thickness to this porridge.

MAKES: 4 servings

PREPARATION TIME: 15 minutes (plus time to refrigerate overnight)

Ingredients

- 2 cups Almond Milk, unsweetened and warmed
- ¼ cup Chia Seeds
- ⅔ cup Old-Fashioned Rolled Oats
- 2 small Bananas, peeled and mashed
- 1 teaspoon Pure Vanilla Extract
- ¼ teaspoon Ground Cinnamon

- 1 cup Raw Buckwheat Groats
- 3 cups Filtered Water
- 2 cups Mixed Fresh Berries (blueberry, blackberry, raspberry etc.)
- 2 tablespoons Almonds, toasted and chopped

Directions

1. In a large bowl, mix together the milk, chia seeds, oats, bananas, vanilla and cinnamon. Cover and refrigerate overnight. In another bowl, soak the buckwheat groats in the water, cover and refrigerate overnight. Remove from refrigerator and rinse well.

2. Divide the oat mixture evenly between serving bowls. Place the buckwheat groats over the oat mixture, top with the berries, sprinkle with the almonds and serve.

SPICED CARROT OATMEAL

This crunchy, creamy and chewy oatmeal is filled with the flavors of carrots, raisins and warm spices. This healthy oatmeal will keep you feeling full for hours.

MAKES: 2 servings
PREPARATION TIME: 10 minutes

COOKING TIME: 10 minutes

Ingredients

- 1¼ cups Unsweetened Almond Milk
- ½ cup Old-Fashioned Rolled Oats
- 1 cup Carrot, peeled and finely grated
- ¼ teaspoon Ground Ginger
- 1 teaspoon Ground Cinnamon
- Pinch of Ground Nutmeg
- Pinch of Ground Cloves
- Pinch of Himalayan Pink Salt
- 2 tablespoons Pure Maple Syrup
- 1 teaspoon Pure Vanilla Extract
- 1 tablespoon Golden Raisins
- 1 tablespoon Almonds, toasted and chopped

Directions

1. In a pan, mix together the milk, oats, carrots and spices on a medium heat. Bring to a boil before reducing the heat to medium-low. Cook, stirring occasionally, for 9 to 10 minutes.

2. Remove from heat and immediately stir in the remaining ingredients before serving.

6

APPETIZERS

FRUIT KABOBS WITH DIP

These kabobs are a beautiful and fun way to serve fruits as a healthy appetizer. Fresh, healthy and delicious fruit are nicely complimented by the creamy and lightly sweet dip.

MAKES: 2 servings

PREPARATION TIME: 20 minutes (plus time to refrigerate)

Ingredients

or Dip:
- 1 cup Raw Cashew nuts, soaked overnight and drained
- ½ cup Fresh Cherries, pitted
- ⅓ cup Almond Milk, unsweetened
- 1 tablespoon Pure Maple Syrup
- 1 teaspoon Vanilla Extract

For Kabobs:
- 1 Orange, peeled, seeded and sectioned
- 1 Apple, peeled, cored and cubed
- 1 Kiwi, peeled and cubed
- 2 Bananas, peeled and sliced
- 6-8 Strawberries, hulled and sliced
- ¼ cup Raspberries

Directions

1. For dip, add all of the ingredients into a blender and pulse until smooth. Transfer the dip into a bowl. Cover and refrigerate for 6 to 8 hours.

2. Thread the fruit pieces onto skewers according to your preference. Serve with the chilled dip.

GRILLED VEGETABLE KABOBS

This is a healthy, simple and delicious way to enjoy vegetables. The tangy and creamy dressing beautifully highlights the flavors of the grilled vegetables.

MAKES: 4 servings
PREPARATION TIME: 15 minutes

COOKING TIME: 15 minutes

Ingredients

For Vegetable Kabobs:
- 2 Yellow Squash, sliced into 1-inch pieces
- 2 Zucchinis, sliced into 1-inch pieces
- 1 Red Bell Pepper, seeded and cut into chunks
- 1 Green Bell Pepper, seeded and cut into chunks
- ½ pound Fresh Mushrooms
- 12 Cherry Tomatoes
- 1 Red Onion, cut into chunks
- 2 tablespoons Almond Butter

For Dressing:
- ½ cup Avocado, peeled, pitted and chopped
- 1 small Garlic Clove, chopped
- ¼ cup Fresh Chives
- 2 tablespoons Fresh Basil Leaves
- 3 tablespoons Fresh Lemon juice
- ¼ cup Almond Butter
- Pinch of Himalayan Pink Salt
- Freshly Ground Black Pepper, as required

Directions

1. Preheat the grill to a medium heat.

2. Thread the vegetables onto the pre-soaked wooden skewers and evenly coat with the almond butter. Grill for about 15 minutes, turning after every 5 minutes.

3. Meanwhile, add all of the dressing ingredients into a food processor and pulse until smooth. Serve the vegetable kabobs with the dressing.

CREAMY MANGO & AVOCADO SALSA

The combination of avocado and mango ensures that this salsa is slightly tangy and creamy in texture. You will find this dish to be heavenly!

MAKES: 2 servings   **PREPARATION TIME:** 10 minutes

Ingredients

- 1 small Ripe Mango, peeled, pitted and chopped
- 1 small Ripe Avocado, peeled, pitted and chopped
- ¼ cup cherry Tomatoes, chopped
- 1 small Red Onion, chopped
- 1 small Jalapeño Pepper, seeded and minced
- 2 tablespoons Almond Butter
- 1 tablespoon Fresh Lime juice
- Pinch of Himalayan Pink Salt
- Freshly Ground Black Pepper, as required
- 2 tablespoons Mint Leaves, freshly chopped

Directions

1. In a large bowl, mix together all of the ingredients.

2. Garnish with mint and serve immediately.

BEAN BRUSCHETTA

This is a delicious appetizer to start off your favorite lavish meal. The balsamic vinegar adds a delicious zip to this easy and delicious bruschetta.

MAKES: 4 servings   **PREPARATION TIME:** 10 minutes

Ingredients

- ¾ cup cooked White Beans
- 1 medium Tomato, chopped
- ½ Garlic Clove, minced
- 2 tablespoons Fresh Scallion, chopped
- 1 tablespoon Balsamic Vinegar

- ⅛ teaspoon Red Pepper Flakes, crushed
- Pinch of Himalayan Pink Salt
- 8 (½-inch thick) toasted Whole Wheat Bread Slices

Directions

1. In a bowl, except for the bread slices, mix together all of the ingredients

2. Place the bean mixture over the bread slices and serve immediately.

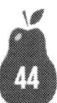

KALE CRACKERS

These crispy but chewy green crackers are perfect as a festive appetizer. They are also a great way to introduce fresh kale into your diet.

MAKES: 4 servings
PREPARATION TIME: 10 minutes

COOKING TIME: 10 minutes

Ingredients

- 3 tablespoons Filtered Water
- ½ cup Fresh Kale, trimmed and chopped
- ½ cup, plus 2 tablespoons, Whole Wheat Flour

- ½ teaspoon Dried Rosemary, crushed
- Pinch of Himalayan Pink Salt
- Pinch of Red Pepper Flakes, crushed
- 2 tablespoons Almond Butter

Directions

1. Preheat the oven to 400 degrees F and line a large baking sheet with parchment paper.

2. In a blender, add the water and kale and pulse until smooth. In a bowl, mix together the flour, rosemary, salt and red pepper flakes. Add the butter and mix until the mixture becomes crumbly. Stir in the kale mixture and mix until a dough forms. Roll the dough to a thinly layer on a floured smooth surface. Cut the rolled dough according to your desired shape.

3. Carefully place the crackers onto the prepared baking sheet and bake for 8 to 10 minutes.

BAKED ONION RINGS

This is one of best and most delicious recipes for crispy and flavorful onion rings. These onion rings will make an excellent addition to your appetizer repertoire.

MAKES: 4 servings
PREPARATION TIME: 15 minutes

COOKING TIME: 18 minutes

Ingredients

- ⅔ cup Whole Wheat Flour
- 2 tablespoons Cornstarch
- ⅔ cup sodium-free Vegetable Broth
- 1 cup Whole Wheat Breadcrumbs
- ½ cup Cornmeal
- ¼ cup Nutritional Yeast

- 1 tablespoon Sesame Seeds
- 2 teaspoons Dried Rosemary, crushed
- 1 large Sweet Onion, sliced into ¾-inch widths

Directions

1. Preheat the oven to 425 degrees F and line a large baking sheet with parchment paper.

2. In a shallow dish, mix together the flour, cornstarch and broth. In another shallow dish, except for the onion rings, mix together the remaining ingredients. Dip the onion rings into the broth mixture then coat with the breadcrumb mixture. Arrange the onion rings on the prepared baking sheet in a single layer.

3. Bake for about 10 minutes before turning and baking for a further 8 minutes. Serve immediately.

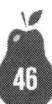

SPICY SWEET POTATO FRIES

This is an easy to cook and absolutely delicious appetizer. Make these fries for your family and you will always get the thumbs up!

MAKES: 4 servings

PREPARATION TIME: 10 minutes

COOKING TIME: 20 minutes

Ingredients

- 3 medium Sweet Potatoes, peeled and sliced into ¾-inch thick wedges
- 1 tablespoon Almond Butter
- ¼ teaspoon Ground Cumin
- ¼ teaspoon Cayenne Pepper
- ¼ teaspoon Red Pepper Flakes, crushed
- Pinch of Himalayan Pink Salt

Directions

1. Preheat the oven to 500 degrees F and line a large baking sheet with parchment paper.

2. Evenly coat the sweet potato wedges with the almond butter and sprinkle with the spices. Arrange the fries on the prepared baking sheet in a single layer. Roast for 10 minutes before turning and roasting for a further 10 minutes.

ROASTED MUSHROOMS

This is an extremely easy yet wonderfully tasting appetizer recipe. Roasting with fresh thyme brings out all the delicious flavors of the mushrooms.

MAKES: 4 servings

COOKING TIME: 30 minutes

PREPARATION TIME: 10 minutes

Ingredients

- 1 pound halved, medium Shiitake Mushrooms
- 1 Garlic Clove, minced
- ¼ cup Thyme Leaves, freshly chopped

- 1 tablespoon Low-Sodium Soy Sauce
- 1 tablespoon Fresh Lime juice
- 1 tablespoon Almond Butter
- 1 cup Fresh Baby Spinach

Directions

1. Preheat the oven to 350 degrees F and line a large baking sheet with parchment paper.

2. Add all ingredients, except for the spinach, to a large bowl and mix well. Transfer the mixture onto the prepared baking sheet and bake for about 30 minutes.

3. Serve the roasted mushrooms over a bed of baby spinach leaves.

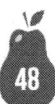

BAKED VEGETABLE BALLS

These surprisingly delicious and nutritious vegetable balls are crispy on the outside yet soft inside.

MAKES: 4 servings
PREPARATION TIME: 10 minutes

COOKING TIME: 25 minutes

Ingredients

- 3 large potatoes, peeled and chopped
- 2 tablespoons sodium-free Vegetable Broth
- 2-3 Garlic Cloves, minced
- 3 cups Fresh Spinach, torn
- 2 tablespoons Scallions, finely chopped
- 1 small Green Pepper, seeded and minced
- 2 tablespoons Fresh Cilantro, chopped
- ½ teaspoon Ground Cumin
- Pinch of Himalayan Pink Salt
- 2 tablespoons Nutritional Yeast

Directions

1. Preheat the oven to 350 degrees F and line a large baking sheet with parchment paper.

2. In a pan of boiling water, add potato and cook for 5 to 6 minutes. Drain well, transfer into a large bowl and mash the potatoes. In a skillet, heat the broth on a medium heat and cook the garlic for about 1 minute before adding the spinach and cooking for a further 2 to 3 minutes. Transfer the spinach mixture into the bowl with the mashed potatoes. Add the remaining ingredients to the bowl and mix well. Make your desired sized balls from the mixture.

3. Arrange the balls on the prepared baking sheet in a single layer and bake for 15 minutes.

SWEET & SOUR CUCUMBER BITES

These pretty little bites are filled with the fresh crunchiness of cucumber coupled with a sweet and sour topping. These are a great and easy appetizer for any gathering.

MAKES: 4 servings   **PREPARATION TIME:** 15 minutes

Ingredients

- 1 large Cucumber, peeled and halved
- 1 Avocado, peeled, pitted and mashed
- 2-3 tablespoons Red Onion, chopped finely
- 2 Medjool Dates, pitted and mashed

- 2 teaspoons Apple Cider Vinegar
- Pinch of Freshly Ground Black Pepper
- ⅛ teaspoon Nutritional Yeast
- ⅛ teaspoon Red Pepper Flakes, crushed

Directions

1. Scoop the seeds from the cucumber and then cut them into 2-inch pieces. Place the cucumber onto a large plate and set aside.

2. In a bowl, mix together the remaining ingredients, except for the red pepper flakes. With a spoon, place the date mixture onto the cucumber pieces. Sprinkle with nutritional yeast and red pepper flakes before serving.

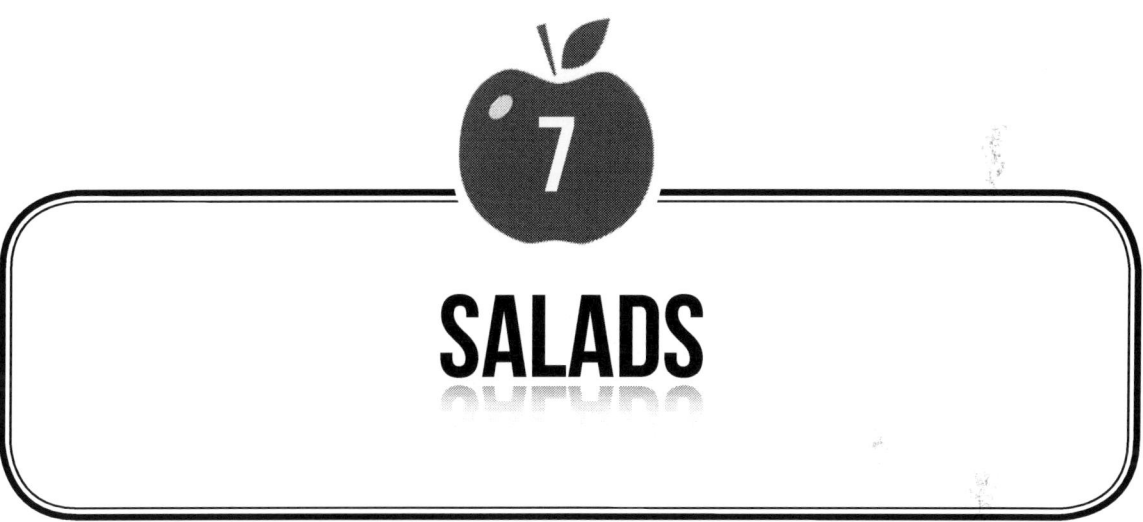

SALADS

CITRUS MIXED FRUIT SALAD

This colorful, refreshing and nutritious summertime salad looks like a beautiful rainbow! The addition of fresh orange in this dish brings a refreshingly tasty touch to this fruit salad.

MAKES: 4 servings

PREPARATION TIME: 15 minutes (plus time to refrigerate)

Ingredients

- 2 Kiwis, peeled and cubed
- 1 medium Mango, peeled, pitted and cubed
- 1 Papaya, peeled, seeded and cubed
- 1 Banana, peeled and sliced
- 1 cup Fresh Strawberries, hulled and halved
- ½ cup Fresh Blueberries
- 2 Oranges, peeled, seeded and sectioned
- 2 tablespoons Fresh Orange juice
- 1 tablespoon Pure Maple Syrup
- ¼ cup chopped Fresh Mint Leaves
- 1 teaspoon Orange Zest, freshly grated

Directions

1. In a large serving bowl, mix together all of the fruits.

2. Mix in the remaining ingredients to the fruit, except for the orange zest. Cover and refrigerate to chill. Top with the orange zest just before serving.

COLORFUL BERRY SALAD

Celebrate family gatherings with this refreshingly delicious berry salad. Lime juice and maple syrup make a slight sweet and tangy dressing for the berries whilst the toasted almonds add a nutty crunch.

MAKES: 4 servings

PREPARATION TIME: 10 minutes

Ingredients

- 1 cup Fresh Strawberries
- 1 cup Fresh Raspberries
- ¾ cup Fresh Blueberries
- ¾ cup Fresh Blackberries
- ¼ cup Fresh Cranberries
- 1 tablespoon Fresh Lime juice
- ½ tablespoon Pure Maple Syrup
- ¼ cup Almonds, toasted and chopped
- 1 tablespoon Mint Leaves, freshly chopped

Directions

1. In a large serving bowl, mix together all of the berries.

2. Add the lime juice and maple syrup and toss to coat. Garnish with the almonds and mint leaves before serving.

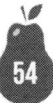

SWEET SPINACH CREAM SPIRALS

This is an easy dish with a sparkling and rich dressing which perfectly balances the spiralized sweet potato and spinach.

MAKES: 2 servings
PREPARATION TIME: 15 minutes

COOKING TIME: 8 minutes

Ingredients

For Dressing:
- ¼ cup (34g) Raw Cashew nuts, soaked for 2 hours and drained
- 1 small Garlic Clove, chopped
- ¼ cup (60ml) unsweetened Almond Milk
- ½ tablespoon Fresh Lime juice
- Himalayan Pink Salt, to taste
- Freshly Ground Black Pepper, to taste

For Vegetables:
- 2 tablespoons Water
- 1 large Sweet Potato, peeled and spiralized
- Himalayan Pink Salt, to taste
- Freshly Ground Black Pepper, to taste
- 1 Garlic Clove, minced
- 3 cups (90g) Fresh Spinach, chopped
- ½ teaspoon Lime Zest, freshly grated

Directions

1. For the dressing, add all of the dressing ingredients into a blender and pulse until smooth.

2. For the vegetables, in a skillet heat 1 tablespoon of water on a medium heat. Add the sweet potato and sprinkle with salt and black pepper, and cook for 6 to 8 minutes. Meanwhile, in another skillet, heat the remaining water on a medium heat. Sauté the garlic for 1 minute. Add the spinach and cook for about 3 minutes. Season with salt and black pepper and remove the pan from the heat.

3. Place the sweet potato and spinach into a large bowl. Combine the dressing with the vegetables and gently mix. Garnish the dish with the lime zest and serve immediately.

APPLE & PEAR SALAD

This is a delicious salad packed with healthy nutrients. The strawberry vinaigrette wonderfully compliments the fruits in a fantastic way!

MAKES: 2 servings

PREPARATION TIME: 15 minutes

Ingredients

For Strawberry Vinaigrette:
- ½ cup Fresh Strawberries, hulled and sliced
- 2 large Medjool Dates, pitted and chopped
- 2 tablespoons Pecans, chopped
- ¼ cup Filtered Water
- ¼ cup Fresh Orange juice
- 1 tablespoon Apple Cider Vinegar

For Salad:
- 1 large Apple, peeled, cored and sliced
- 1 large Pear, peeled, cored and sliced
- 4 cups Fresh Mixed Greens
- 2 tablespoons Pumpkin Seeds, toasted

Directions

1. In a blender, add all of the vinaigrette ingredients and pulse until smooth.

2. In a large salad bowl, mix together the fruits and greens. Pour the vinaigrette over the salad and toss to coat well. Top with the pumpkin seeds and serve.

MIXED CITRUS SALAD

This refreshingly tangy and easily prepared salad is packed with the goodness of citrus fruit.

MAKES: 4 servings

PREPARATION TIME: 15 minutes (plus time to refrigerate)

Ingredients

- 1 Naval Orange, peeled, seeded and sectioned
- 1 Mandarin Orange, peeled, seeded and sectioned
- 2 Grape Fruits, peeled, seeded and sectioned
- ½ tablespoon Pure Maple Syrup
- 1 tablespoon Mint Leaves, freshly chopped
- 1 teaspoon Orange Zest, freshly grated

Directions

1. In a large serving bowl, mix together all of the ingredients, except for the orange zest. Cover and refrigerate to chill before serving.

2. Garnish with the orange zest and serve.

STRAWBERRY SPINACH SALAD

This fresh salad is ideal for a lovely summer's day and may brighten your dinner table. This salad is bound to become a family favorite.

MAKES: 2 servings   **PREPARATION TIME:** 15 minutes

Ingredients

For Vinaigrette:
- 1 small Garlic Clove, minced
- ¼ teaspoon Fresh Dill Weed
- ½ tablespoon Apple Cider Vinegar
- 1 tablespoon Fresh Lime juice
- 1 tablespoon Pure Maple Syrup
- Pinch of Freshly Ground Black Pepper

For Salad:
- 1 cup Fresh Strawberries, hulled and sliced
- 4 cups Fresh Baby Spinach
- 1 Scallion, chopped
- 1 tablespoon Walnuts, chopped

Directions

1. In a small bowl, mix together the garlic, dill weed, vinegar, lime juice, maple syrup and black pepper.

2. In a large salad bowl, mix together the strawberries, spinach and scallion. Pour the vinaigrette over the salad and toss to coat well. Top with the walnuts and serve.

CRUNCHY BRUSSELS SPROUT SALAD

This salad is nutritious, crunchy and vibrant. It has a combination of healthy and delicious ingredients.

MAKES: 4 servings   **PREPARATION TIME:** 15 minutes

Ingredients

- 2 medium Carrots, peeled and shredded
- 1½ cups Brussels Sprouts, trimmed and chopped
- 1 Celery Stalk, chopped
- 1 Apple, cored and chopped
- 1 teaspoon Parsley Leaves, freshly chopped

- ¼ cup Golden Raisins
- ¼ cup Sunflower Seeds
- 3 tablespoons Fresh Lime juice
- 1 teaspoon Pure Maple Syrup
- Pinch of Freshly Ground Black Pepper
- ¼ teaspoon Ground Cinnamon

Directions

1. In a large serving bowl, except for the cinnamon, mix together all of the salad ingredients.

2. Sprinkle with the ground cinnamon and serve.

CUCUMBER MINT SALAD

This is a delicious and healthy addition to your salad menu list. This recipe is a combination of a few simple ingredients which makes this salad really memorable.

MAKES: 4 servings

PREPARATION TIME: 10 minutes (plus time to refrigerate)

Ingredients

- 2 large English Cucumbers, sliced thinly
- Pinch of Pink Himalayan Salt
- 2 tablespoons Pure Maple Syrup
- ¼ cup Fresh Lime juice
- Pinch of Freshly Ground Black Pepper
- 2 tablespoons Mint Leaves, freshly chopped

Directions

1. In a large colander, place the cucumber and sprinkle with the salt. Set aside for at least 10 to 15 minutes before patting dry the cucumber slices with a paper towel. Transfer the cucumber into a large serving bowl.

2. Meanwhile, in a small bowl mix together the remaining ingredients. Pour the dressing over the cucumber and gently stir to mix. Cover and refrigerate to chill before serving.

CABBAGE & CARROT SALAD

This crunchy cabbage and carrot salad is a fantastically healthy dish for all meals. It is so delicious that your family may ask for it time and again.

MAKES: 4 servings　　　　　　　　**PREPARATION TIME:** 15 minutes

Ingredients

For Dressing:
- 1 Garlic Clove, minced
- ¼ cup Fresh Cilantro Leaves, chopped
- 2 tablespoons Almond Butter
- 2 tablespoons Fresh Lime juice
- Pinch of Freshly Ground Black Pepper

For Salad:
- 3 cups Purple Cabbage, roughly chopped
- 3 cups Green Cabbage, roughly chopped
- 2 Carrots, peeled and shredded
- 2 Celery Stalks, chopped
- 3 tablespoons Sesame Seeds

Directions

1. In a blender, add all of the vinaigrette ingredients and pulse until smooth.

2. In a large salad bowl, mix together the cabbage, carrots and celery. Pour the dressing over the salad and toss to coat well. Top with the sesame seeds and serve.

MIXED TOMATO AVOCADO SALAD

This refreshing and healthy salad is a great hit as a cooling accompaniment to any kind of savory meal.

MAKES: 2 servings   **PREPARATION TIME:** 15 minutes

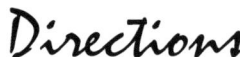 *Ingredients*

- 1 Avocado, peeled, pitted and chopped
- 1 cup Cherry Tomatoes, halved
- 1 cup Grape Tomatoes, halved
- 1 tablespoon Red Onion, chopped
- 1 small Garlic Clove, minced

- 3 tablespoons Mint Leaves, freshly chopped
- 1 tablespoon Fresh Lime juice
- Pinch of Freshly Ground Black Pepper

Directions

1. Add all of the ingredients into a large serving bowl and toss to coat well.

2. Serve immediately.

ROASTED SWEET POTATO VEGGIE SALAD

This is a hearty and delicious vegetable salad. The roasted sweet potato and other fresh vegetables pair nicely with the sweet and tangy dressing.

MAKES: 4 servings
PREPARATION TIME: 15 minutes

COOKING TIME: 30 minutes

Ingredients

For Salad:
- 1 large Sweet Potato, peeled and cut into bite sized pieces
- 1 tablespoon Almond Butter
- 1 medium Carrot, peeled and chopped
- 1 Orange Bell Pepper, seeded and chopped
- 1 small Cucumber, chopped
- 1 small Red Onion, chopped
- 1 Scallion, chopped
- ¼ cup Fresh Parsley Leaves, chopped
- ½ cup Walnuts, toasted and chopped

For Dressing:
- ¼ cup Almond Butter
- 1 small Garlic Clove, chopped
- 2 tablespoons Low-Sodium Soy Sauce
- 2 tablespoons Fresh Lemon juice
- 2 teaspoons Pure Maple Syrup
- 2 tablespoons Filtered Water

Directions

1. Preheat the oven to 400 degrees F and line a roasting dish with parchment paper. Place the sweet potato into the prepared roasting pan and coat with the almond butter. Roast for 15 minutes before turning the potatoes and roasting for another 15 minutes. Remove the dish from the oven and transfer the potatoes into a large bowl. Let them cool before mixing in the remaining vegetables.

2. In a blender, add all of the dressing ingredients and pulse until smooth. Pour the salad dressing over the salad and toss to coat.

3. Top with the parsley and walnuts before serving.

CORN & BASIL SALAD

This is an easy and crunchy summer salad which is ideal for family meals and potlucks. The natural sweetness of the corn compliments nicely with acidity of the vinegar.

MAKES: 4 servings
PREPARATION TIME: 15 minutes

COOKING TIME: 4 minutes

Ingredients

- 5 Corn Ears, husked
- ½ cup Cherry Tomatoes, halved
- ½ cup Red Onion, chopped
- 2 scallions (Green part), chopped
- ½ cup Fresh Basil Leaves, chopped
- 2 tablespoons Balsamic Vinegar
- Pinch of Pink Himalayan Salt
- Freshly Ground Black Pepper, to taste

Directions

1. In a large pan of boiling water, add the corn ears and cook for 3 to 4 minutes. Drain the corn ears and immediately place them into a bowl of ice water. With a sharp knife, cut off the kernels. Transfer the kernels into a large serving bowl.

2. Add all of the remaining ingredients and toss to coat well before serving.

SPICY POTATO BEAN SALAD

This is an incredibly delicious bean and potato salad which is ideal for all types of gatherings. The combination of the tangy yogurt dressing and spices makes this a wonderfully delicious salad.

MAKES: 4 servings   **PREPARATION TIME:** 15 minutes

Ingredients

For Spicy Dressing:
- 1 cup plain Soy Yogurt
- 1 small Garlic Clove, minced
- ¼ cup Fresh Basil Leaves, chopped
- ½ teaspoon Ground Coriander
- 1 teaspoon Ground Cumin
- ½ teaspoon Red Pepper Flakes, crushed
- 2 tablespoons Fresh Lime juice

For Salad:
- 1 cup cooked Garbanzo Beans
- 1 cupcooked Red Kidney Beans
- 2 cupscooked Potatoes, peeled and cubed
- ½ cup Fresh Tomato, chopped
- ½ cup Cucumber, chopped
- ¼ cup Red Onion, chopped

Directions

1. In a blender, add all of the dressing ingredients and pulse until smooth.

2. In a large salad bowl, mix together all of the salad ingredients. Pour the dressing over the salad and toss to coat well before serving immediately.

QUINOA BEAN SALAD

This is a perfect and nutritious salad for those special occasions and potlucks. The quinoa compliments nicely with the salad ingredients and the tangy dressing.

MAKES: 4 servings   **PREPARATION TIME:** 15 minutes

Ingredients

For Dressing:
- 1 Garlic Clove, minced
- 1 Jalapeño Pepper, seeded and chopped
- 1½ tablespoons no-sodium Vegetable Broth
- 2 tablespoons Fresh Lime juice

For Salad:
- 1 cup cooked Quinoa
- 1 cup cooked Black Beans
- ½ cup cooked Corn
- 1 small Avocado, peeled, pitted and chopped
- 1 small Cucumber, peeled, seeded and chopped
- 1 medium Fresh Tomato, chopped
- ¼ cup Scallion, chopped
- ½ cu Fresh Parsley, chopped

Directions

1. In a blender, add all of the dressing ingredients and pulse until smooth.

2. In a large salad bowl, mix together all of the salad ingredients. Pour the dressing over the salad, toss to coat well and serve immediately.

HERBED COUSCOUS SALAD

This is a simple and delicious couscous salad with fresh herbs and vegetables. This salad may become a favorite salad on your menu list.

MAKES: 2 servings
PREPARATION TIME: 15 minutes

COOKING TIME: 3 minutes

Ingredients

For Couscous:
- ¾ cup Dry Whole Wheat Couscous
- 1 cup Low-Sodium Vegetable Broth
- 1 tablespoon Almond Butter
- 2 Fresh ParsleyStems
- 1 teaspoon Lemon Zest
- Pinch of Red Chili Powder
- 2 Scallions, chopped
- 2 tablespoons Parsley Leaves, freshly chopped

For Salad:
- 1 medium Cucumber, peeled, seeded and chopped
- 1½ cups Grape Tomatoes, halved
- 1 tablespoon Fresh Lemon juice
- ¼ cup Fresh MintLeaves, chopped

Directions

1. In a large bowl, place the couscous and set aside. In a pan, add the broth, butter, parsley stems, lemon zest and chili powder. Bring to a boil on a high heat for 2 to 3 minutes. Pour the boiling broth solution over the couscous. Cover the bowl and set aside for at least 5 minutes. Remove the cover and discard the parsley stem and lemon zest. With a fork, fluff the couscous. Add the scallion and parsley leaves and mix.

2. In another bowl, mix together all of the salad ingredients. Add the cucumber mixture to the bowl with the couscous. Stir to mix well before serving immediately.

CREAMY PASTA SALAD

This recipe makes a quick, easy and delicious pasta salad. The dressing with this salad adds a wonderfully delicious creamy texture to the pasta and vegetables.

MAKES: 4 servings

PREPARATION TIME: 15 minutes

COOKING TIME: 10 minutes

Ingredients

For Pasta Salad:
- 1 cup Whole Wheat Pasta (of your choice)
- ½ Orange Bell Pepper, seeded and chopped
- ½ Red Bell Pepper, seeded and chopped
- 2 Scallions, chopped
- ½ cup Fresh Basil Leaves, chopped

For Creamy Dressing:
- 2-3 Garlic Cloves, minced
- ½ cup no-sodium Vegetable Broth
- 2 tablespoons Almond Butter
- 2 tablespoons Low-Sodium Soy Sauce
- 1 teaspoon Red Pepper Flakes, crushed

Directions

1. In a pan of boiling water, cook the pasta for 8 to 10 minutes. Drain and rinse with cold water before transferring the pasta into a large serving bowl. Mix the remaining salad ingredients with the pasta.

2. In another bowl, beat together all of the dressing ingredients. Pour the dressing over the salad, toss to coat well and serve immediately.

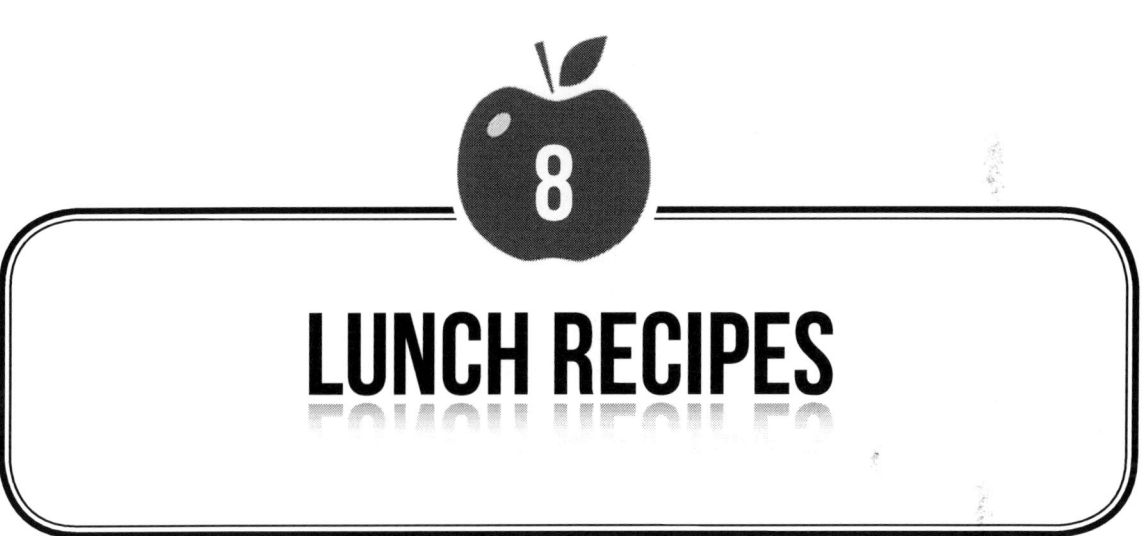

LUNCH RECIPES

QUINOA BEAN WRAPS

This is an awesome recipe for mouthwatering wraps! These wraps are easy to make and assemble and make a wonderfully light, delicious and healthy lunch.

MAKES: 4 servings

PREPARATION TIME: 15 minutes

COOKING TIME: 3 minutes

Ingredients

- 1 cup cooked Navy Beans
- 1½ cups cooked Quinoa
- ½ cup Non-Fat, Low-Sodium Salsa
- 1 teaspoon Low-Sodium Hot Sauce
- Pinch of Freshly Ground Black Pepper
- 4 large Iceberg Lettuce Leaves

- ½ cup Red Onion, chopped
- ½ cup Plum Tomatoes, chopped
- 1 Jalapeño Pepper, seeded and chopped
- 1 medium Avocado, peeled, pitted and sliced

Directions

1. In a large skillet on a medium-low heat, add the beans, quinoa, salsa, hot sauce and black pepper. Cook for 2 to 3 minutes or until heated through completely. Transfer the mixture into a bowl.

2. Arrange the lettuce leaves on large plates and evenly place the bean mixture onto each lettuce leaf. Top with the remaining ingredients and serve immediately.

SWEET & SOUR VEGETABLE ROLLS

These rolls are quick to prepare, delicious, and they are also packed with an incredibly healthy vegetable filling. The sweet and sour sauce is perfect for these fresh vegetable rolls.

MAKES: 4 servings   **PREPARATION TIME:** 20 minutes

Ingredients

For Sweet & Sour Sauce:
- ¼ teaspoon Fresh Ginger, peeled and chopped
- 3 small Garlic Cloves, chopped
- 1 bunch Fresh Cilantro, chopped
- ½ cup Almond Butter
- ¼ cup Pure Maple Syrup
- 1 tablespoon Low-Sodium Soy Sauce
- 2 tablespoons Balsamic Vinegar

For Rolls:
- 2 large Carrots, peeled and thinly sliced
- 2 Cucumbers, peeled, seeded and thinly sliced
- 1 large Yellow Bell Pepper, seeded and sliced thinly
- 1 large Avocado, peeled, pitted and sliced
- 2 tablespoons minced Cilantro Leaves
- 1 tablespoon Low-Sodium Soy Sauce
- 4 large Whole Collard Green Leaves

Directions

1. For the sauce, add all of the ingredients into a blender and pulse until smooth. Transfer the sauce into a bowl and set aside.

2. For the rolls, in a large bowl mix together all of the ingredients, except for the collard greens. Arrange the collard green leaves on large plates and evenly place the vegetable mixture onto each leaf. Roll the leaves and serve with the sauce.

MUSHROOM TORTILLA WRAPS

This is a great and tasty way to use mushrooms. These tortilla wraps, not only being a great addition to your lunch time menu, but are also healthy and delicious.

MAKES: 2 servings

PREPARATION TIME: 10 minutes (plus time to marinate)

COOKING TIME: 10 minutes

Ingredients

- 2 tablespoons Fresh Lime juice
- 3 tablespoons Fresh Orange juice
- 2 tablespoons Low-Sodium Soy Sauce
- ¼ teaspoon Dried Oregano, crushed
- ¼ teaspoon Dried Oregano, crushed
- ¼ teaspoon Dried Thyme, crushed
- 1 teaspoon Ground Cumin
- 1 teaspoon Smoked Paprika
- ½ teaspoon Red Pepper Flakes, crushed

- 4 Portobello Mushrooms, sliced into 1-inch pieces
- 2 tablespoons Sodium free Vegetable Broth
- ½ Red Onion, chopped
- 1 small Fresh Tomato, chopped
- ¼ cup Cilantro Leaves, freshly chopped
- 2 (10-inch) warmed Whole Grain Tortillas
- 2 tablespoons Low-Sodium Soy Sauce

Directions

1. In a large bowl, mix together the citrus juices, soy sauce, herbs and spices. Add the mushrooms and generously coat with the mixture. Cover and refrigerate for at least 3 to 4 hours. In a nonstick skillet, heat the broth on medium heat. Add the mushrooms with marinade and sauté for 8 to 10 minutes. Remove from the heat and transfer into a bowl.

2. Meanwhile, in a bowl mix together the onion, tomato, cilantro and lime juice. Arrange the warmed tortillas on large plates. Place the mushrooms onto each tortilla and top with the onion mixture. Roll the tortillas, cut from the center and serve.

BEAN VEGETABLE SANDWICHES

These sandwiches are light yet super delicious for a lunch recipe. They are also perfect for a kid's school lunch box.

MAKES: 2 servings   **PREPARATION TIME:** 15 minutes

Ingredients

- 1¼ cups cooked Navy Beans
- 1 tablespoon Fresh Lime juice
- Pinch of Freshly Ground Black Pepper
- 4 Whole Wheat Bread Slices
- 4 Tomato Slices
- ½ Avocado, peeled, pitted and sliced thinly
- ½ cup Baby Spinach

Directions

1. In a food processor, add the beans, lemon juice and black pepper and pulse until smooth before transferring into a bowl.

2. Place 2 bread slices on serving plates and spread the bean mixture evenly over each slice. Top with tomato, avocado and spinach before covering with the remaining 2 slices. With a sharp knife, cut the sandwiches into triangles and serve.

BAKED SPICY BEAN BURGERS

These tasty burgers, filled with healthy nutrients, will be a treat for the whole family. These burgers taste so great even meat-lovers will find them irresistible!

MAKES: 4 servings
PREPARATION TIME: 15 minutes

COOKING TIME: 40 minutes

Ingredients

For Patties:
- ¼ cup Warm Filtered Water
- 1¼ tablespoons Flax Seeds
- 1 tablespoon sodium-free Vegetable Broth
- ¼ cup White Onion, chopped
- 1 small Garlic Clove, minced
- ½ cup Carrot, peeled and grated
- 2 tablespoons minced Cilantro Leaves
- ½ cup cooked Chickpeas, mashed
- ½ cup Almond Flour
- ¾ cup Whole Wheat Bread Crumbs
- ¼ cup Sunflower Seeds, toasted and chopped

- 3 tablespoons Almonds, toasted and chopped
- ½ tablespoon Low-Sodium Soy Sauce
- ¼ teaspoon Dried Rosemary, crushed
- ¼ teaspoon Dried Oregano, crushed
- ½ teaspoon Ground Cumin
- ¼ teaspoon Red Pepper Flakes, crushed
- Pinch of Cayenne Pepper

For Burgers:
- 4 Whole Wheat Buns, split and toasted
- 4 Lettuce Leaves
- 4 large Tomato Slices

Directions

1. Preheat the oven to 350 degrees F and line a baking sheet with parchment paper.

2. In a large bowl, mix the water and flax seeds together and set aside for at least 10 minutes. Meanwhile, in a skillet heat the broth on a medium heat. Sauté the onion and garlic for 8 to 10 minutes. Transfer the onion mixture into the bowl with the flax seed mixture. Add the remaining ingredients and mix well. Make 4 equal sized patties from the mixture. Arrange the patties on the prepared baking sheet in a single layer and bake for about 15 minutes. Turn the patties and bake for a further 15 minutes.

3. Arrange the bottom piece of each bun on serving plates. Place the lettuce leaves on each bun and arrange the patties over the lettuce. Top with the tomato slices before covering with the other part of each bun and serve.

BAKED VEGETABLE PANCAKES

This is a warming holiday meal for all seasons. It makes a healthy, delicious and crispy meal for lunch. You will find that your kids will love to eat these pancakes!

MAKES: 2 servings
PREPARATION TIME: 10 minutes

COOKING TIME: 16 minutes

Ingredients

- 3 tablespoons Filtered Water
- 1 tablespoon Ground Flax Seeds
- 1 cup Russet Potato, peeled and grated finely
- 1 cup Sweet Potato, peeled and grated finely
- 1 small Garlic Clove, minced
- 1 tablespoon Scallion, minced
- ½ teaspoon Cilantro Leaves, freshly minced
- ¼ cup Spelt Flour
- ¼ teaspoon Ground Cumin
- ⅛ teaspoon Smoked Paprika
- ⅛ teaspoon Cayenne Pepper
- Pinch of Pink Himalayan Salt

Directions

1. Preheat the oven to 400 degrees F and line a baking sheet with parchment paper.

2. In a large bowl, mix together the water and flax seeds. Add the remaining ingredients and mix until thoroughly combined. Place ¼ cup of the potato mixture onto the prepared baking sheet and, with your hands, flatten slightly. Repeat with remaining mixture. Bake for about 16 minutes, turning once after 8 minutes.

TOFU & KALE LASAGNA

This hearty and flavorful recipe makes a great lasagna which is ideal for lunch. This dish is packed with the filling of tofu, kale and tomato sauce, something the whole family will enjoy.

MAKES: 4 servings

PREPARATION TIME: 15 minutes

COOKING TIME: 32 minutes

Ingredients

- 3 cups Fresh Kale, trimmed and chopped
- 2-3 tablespoons Fresh Oregano Leaves
- 1 Garlic Clove, chopped
- 2 pounds Silken Tofu, pressed
- ¼ cup Soy Milk
- 2 tablespoons Fresh Lime juice
- 4 cups Low-Sodium Tomato Sauce
- ½ pound Whole Wheat Lasagna Noodles, cooked as per the package instructions

Directions

1. Preheat the oven to 350 degrees F. In a pan of boiling water add the kale and cook for 1 to 2 minutes. Drain and squeeze well before setting aside. In a blender, add the oregano, garlic, tofu, soy milk and lime juice and pulse until smooth. Divide the lasagna noodles in three parts.

2. Spread a thin layer of tomato sauce in a 9x13-inch baking dish. Place 1 part of noodles over the tomato sauce. Top with half of the tofu mixture and then spinach evenly. Top with half of the tomato sauce. Repeat the layer of noodles, tofu mixture and spinach. Top with the remaining noodles and spread the remaining sauce over noodles.

3. Bake for 25 to 30 minutes or until the top becomes bubbly.

MACARONI WITH SQUASH SAUCE

This meal, a hit recipe for lunchtime, is simply delicious and filling. Surely you will love the combination of macaroni with squash sauce.

MAKES: 4 servings
PREPARATION TIME: 15 minutes

COOKING TIME: 43 minutes

Ingredients

- 1 (3½-pound) peeled, seeded and diced Butternut Squash
- 1 tablespoon Almond Butter
- ¼ cup Raw Cashews, soaked overnight and drained
- 1-2 Garlic Cloves, chopped
- 1 tablespoon Fresh Lime juice
- 1 tablespoon Low-Sodium Hot Sauce
- ½-¾ cup Filtered Water

- 2 tablespoons Nutritional Yeast
- ¼ teaspoon Red Pepper Flakes, crushed
- ¼ teaspoon Smoked Paprika
- Pinch of Freshly Ground Black Pepper
- 2 cups Whole Grain Macaroni, cooked according to package directions

Directions

1. Preheat the oven to 425 degrees F and line a large baking dish with parchment paper. Arrange the squash on the prepared baking dish. Coat with the almond butter and roast for about 20 minutes. Turn the squash and roast for a further 15 to 20 minutes. Remove the dish from the oven and set aside to cool. In a blender, add the roasted squash and remaining ingredients, except for the macaroni, and pulse until smooth.

2. In a skillet, add the squash sauce and pasta on a medium heat. Cook for 2 to 3 minutes, or until heated before serving.

GRILLED TOFU WITH SPINACH SAUCE

This recipe is a great and delicious way of cooking tofu. The grilled spicy tofu is wonderfully dressed up in a fantastic spinach sauce. This is guaranteed to be loved by all tofu lovers.

MAKES: 2 servings

COOKING TIME: 8 minutes

PREPARATION TIME: 15 minutes (plus time to marinate)

Ingredients

For Grilled Tofu:
- 2 small Garlic Cloves, minced
- ½ Jalapeño Pepper, seeded and chopped
- ¼ cup Fresh Lemon juice
- 2 tablespoons Low-Sodium Soy Sauce
- 1 tablespoon Pure Maple Syrup
- Freshly Ground Black Pepper, to taste
- 1 (8-ounce) package Extra Firm Tofu, drained, pressed and cut into 4 slices

For Spinach Sauce:
- ½ cup Fresh Spinach, chopped
- ¼ cup Basil Leaves, freshly chopped
- 1 small Garlic Clove, chopped
- 2 tablespoons Almond Milk
- 2 tablespoons Fresh Lemon juice
- Pinch of Pink Himalayan Salt
- Pinch of Freshly Ground Black Pepper

Directions

1. For the tofu, mix all of the ingredients into a large bowl. Cover and refrigerate to marinate for at least 4 hours.

2. In a food processor, add all of the sauce ingredients and pulse until smooth before setting aside.

3. Preheat the grill to a medium heat. Grill the tofu for about 8 minutes, turning once after 4 minutes. Transfer the tofu onto a serving plate. Add the spinach sauce and gently mix with the tofu before serving immediately.

CURRIED TOFU & VEGETABLES

This is a delicious vegan recipe. The combination of tofu and vegetables with curry powder make this curry really hearty and filling.

MAKES: 4 servings
PREPARATION TIME: 15 minutes

COOKING TIME: 35 minutes

Ingredients

- 1½ cups Onion, chopped
- 2 Garlic Cloves, chopped
- 2 teaspoons Fresh Ginger, chopped
- 1 Jalapeño Pepper, chopped
- 1 (8-ounce) package Firm Tofu
- 3 tablespoons Sodium free Vegetable Broth
- 3 teaspoons Curry Powder

- 1½ cups unsweetened Soy Milk or Almond Milk
- 1 cup Filtered Water
- 1¼ cups carrot, peeled and sliced diagonally into ¼-inch pieces
- 1½ cups Tomato, sliced into wedges
- 3 cups Broccoli, cut into florets

Directions

1. In a food processor, add the onion, garlic, ginger and jalapeño and pulse until smooth. Set aside. Cube the tofu and add it to a nonstick skillet heated on a medium heat, and cook for 5 minutes. Turn and cook for 5 minutes more. Transfer the tofu onto a plate and set aside.

2. In the same skillet, heat the broth on a medium heat. Add the onion paste and sauté for 4 to 5 minutes. Add the curry powder, soy milk, water and carrot and bring to a boil before reducing the heat, covering and simmering for about 10 minutes. Add the tofu, tomatoes and broccoli and simmer for a further 5 to 10 minutes.

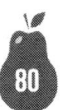

QUINOA WITH ROASTED BEANS & CAULIFLOWER

This is a healthy dish which has a deliciously tangy cashew nut sauce.

MAKES: 2 servings
PREPARATION TIME: 15 minutes

COOKING TIME: 30 minutes

Ingredients

For Quinoa Bowl:
- 3 cups Cauliflower, cut into bite size pieces
- 1 cup cooked Garbanzo Beans
- 1 tablespoon Almond Butter
- 1 tablespoon Low-Sodium Hot Sauce
- Freshly Ground Black Pepper, to taste
- 2 cups Cooked Quinoa

For Cashew Sauce:
- ½ cup Raw Cashew nuts, soaked for 2 hours and drained
- 1 Garlic Clove, chopped
- 2 tablespoons Fresh Basil Leaves
- 3 tablespoons Nutritional Yeast
- 2 tablespoons Fresh Lime juice
- 3 tablespoons Filtered Water

Directions

1. Preheat the oven to 400 degrees F and line a large baking sheet with parchment paper. Place all of the ingredients, except for the quinoa, in the prepared baking sheet and stir to coat well. Roast for about 15 minutes before turning the bean mixture and roasting for a further 15 minutes. Transfer the bean mixture into a bowl. Add the quinoa and mix.

2. Meanwhile, in a blender add all of the sauce ingredients and pulse until smooth. Pour the sauce over the quinoa mixture and serve.

SAUTÉED GREENS & BELL PEPPER

This is one of the simplest, quickest and tastiest dishes for lunch. This dish is packed with sharply flavored and nutritionally-rich fresh greens which nicely complement with the soy sauce and vinegar.

MAKES: 2 servings

COOKING TIME: 10 minutes

PREPARATION TIME: 10 minutes

Ingredients

- ¼ cup sodium-free Vegetable Broth
- 1 small White Onion, chopped
- 2-3 Garlic Cloves, minced
- 1 tablespoon Fresh Ginger, grated
- 1 Jalapeño Pepper, seeded and chopped
- ½ pound Collard Greens, chopped
- ½ pound Mustard Greens, chopped
- 1 tablespoon Balsamic Vinegar
- 1 tablespoon Low-Sodium Soy Sauce
- ½ teaspoon Nutritional Yeast

Directions

1. In a large skillet, heat 2 tablespoons of the broth on a medium heat. Sauté the onion for 3 to 4 minutes before adding the garlic, ginger and jalapeño and sautéing for 1 minute more. Add the greens, vinegar, soy sauce and remaining broth, and sauté for a further 4 to 5 minutes.

2. Sprinkle with nutritional yeast and serve.

SPICED CAULIFLOWER & POTATO

This simple recipe, having a mind blowing combination of delicious ingredients, will leave you amazed with its rich flavors.

MAKES: 4 servings
PREPARATION TIME: 15 minutes

COOKING TIME: 45 minutes

Ingredients

- 3 tablespoons sodium-free Vegetable Broth
- 1 medium White Onion, chopped
- 3 Garlic Cloves, minced
- ½ tablespoon Fresh Ginger, grated
- 1 tablespoon Ground Cumin
- ½ tablespoon Ground Cilantro
- ½ teaspoon Red Pepper Flakes, crushed
- 3 cups Plum Tomatoes, finely chopped

- 3 cups Potatoes, peeled and cubed
- ¾ cup unsweetened Almond Milk
- ½ small Head Cauliflower, cut into large bite size pieces
- 2 cups Fresh Spinach, torn
- 1½ cups cooked Garbanzo Beans
- Pinch of Pink Himalayan Salt
- 2 tablespoons Parsley Leaves, freshly chopped

Directions

1. In a large pan, heat the broth on a medium-high heat. Sauté the onion for 8 to 10 minutes before sautéing the garlic, ginger and spices for 1 minute more. Add the plum tomatoes and cook, stirring, for a further minute. Add the potatoes and almond milk and bring to a boil before reducing the heat, covering and simmering for 15 to 20 minutes more.

2. Stir in the cauliflower and simmer for 10 minutes. Stir in the spinach and beans and simmer for a further 2 to 3 minutes. Season with salt and garnish with parsley before serving.

STIR-COOKED GREEN BEANS

These stir-cooked green beans are perfect for alone or for serving with everyday meals, and are prepared in minutes. Garlic adds a wonderful flavour to the beans. Garnish with lime wedges.

Serves: 2

Cooking Time: 9 minutes

Prep Time: 10 minutes

Ingredients

- ½ pound Fresh Green Beans, trimmed
- ½ tablespoon Balsamic Vinegar
- 1 tablespoon Low-sodium Soy Sauce
- 2 tablespoons sodium-free Vegetable Broth
- 1 teaspoon Garlic, minced
- Freshly Ground Black Pepper, to taste

Directions

1. In a pan of boiling water, add the beans and cook for about 5 minutes before draining.

2. In a bowl, mix together the soy sauce and vinegar. Leave aside.

3. In a skillet, heat the 2 tablespoon of vegetable broth on a medium heat. Sauté the garlic for 1 minute. Add the beans and the vinegar mixture. Stir for about 2 to 3 minutes.

4. Season with black pepper and serve.

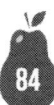

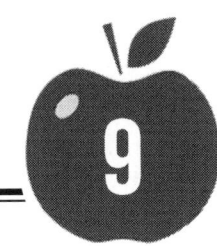

SOUP RECIPES

CHICKPEA MUSHROOM SOUP

This easily prepared soup is amazingly tasty, as well as very healthy. It tastes great on the day made, and even better the day after.

Servings: 2
Preparation Time: 10 minutes

Cooking Time: 27 minutes

Ingredients

- 1 tablespoon Water
- 1 small Garlic Clove, chopped
- ½ cup Onion, chopped
- ½ Green Bell Pepper, chopped
- 3 Button Mushrooms, chopped
- Pinch of Red Pepper Flakes, crushed
- Pinch of Paprika
- ¼ teaspoon Dried Thyme, crushed
- ¼ teaspoon Dried Oregano, crushed

- 1 cup (240ml)Tomato Paste
- 2 cups (480ml) no-sodium Vegetable Broth
- 1 cup Cooked Chickpeas
- Himalayan Salt, to taste (optional)
- Freshly Ground Black pepper, to taste
- ½ tablespoon Fresh Lemon juice

Directions

1. Heat the water in a large soup pan over a medium heat. Add the garlic, onion, bell pepper, mushrooms, spices and herbs, and sauté for about 5 minutes.

2. Add the tomato paste and cook for a further 1 to 2 minutes. Add the broth and chickpeas, and bring to the boil. Cover and, on a low heat, simmer for 20 minutes.

3. Stir in the lemon juice and season with Himalayan salt and black pepper.

4. Serve hot.

LENTIL VEGGIE SOUP

Lentils and carrots, cooked with spices, make this soup flavorful and delicious. Serve garnished with a drizzle of lime juice.

Serves: 2
Preparation Time: 10 minutes

Cooking Time: 42 minutes

Ingredients

- 1 tablespoon Water
- ¼ cup Onion, chopped
- ¼ cup Celery, chopped
- ¼ Carrot, peeled and chopped
- 1 small Tomato, chopped finely
- 4 cups no-sodium Vegetable Broth
- ¾ cup tomatoes, chopped finely

- ½ cup Lentils
- ¼ teaspoon Ground Cumin
- ¼ teaspoon Ground Cilantro
- Himalayan Salt, to taste
- Freshly Ground Black pepper, to taste

Directions

1. Heat the water in a large soup pan over a medium heat. Add the onion, celery and carrot, and sauté for 5 to 7 minutes. Add the broth, tomato, lentils, cumin, cilantro and seasonings before bringing the pan to the boil.

2. Reduce the heat to low and simmer for 30 to 35 minutes. With a stick blender, puree the soup to your liking.

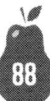

SQUASH MIX SOUP

This healthy soup is packed full of protein. The aroma of the spices will bring everyone to the table at once! Top with freshly grated lemon zest.

Serves: 2

Preparation Time: 20 minutes

Cooking Time: 30 minutes

Ingredients

- 1 tablespoon Water
- ½ small Onion, chopped
- 2 Garlic Cloves, chopped
- ½ small Carrot, peeled and chopped
- ¼ cup Celery, chopped
- ½ small Red Bell Pepper, seeded and chopped
- ¼ teaspoon Ground Cumin
- ¼ teaspoon Ground Cilantro
- ½ teaspoon Red Pepper Flakes, crushed

- ½ teaspoon Chili Powder
- 1 cup Tomatoes, chopped finely
- ½ cup (180ml) Tomato Paste
- 4 cups no-sodium Chicken Broth
- ¼ cup Dried Green Lentils
- ½ cup Cooked Navy Beans
- ½ cup Cooked Cannellini Beans
- 1 small Yellow Squash, chopped
- 1 small Summer Squash, chopped
- Himalayan Salt, to taste
- Freshly Ground Black pepper, to taste

Directions

1. Heat the water in a large soup pan over a medium heat. Add the garlic, onion, celery, carrot, and bell pepper, and sauté for 10 minutes. Add the spices and sauté for a further 2 minutes. Add the tomato paste and tomatoes, cooking for a further 3 minutes.

2. Add the broth, lentils and beans to the pan, and bring to the boil. Stir in the squashes.

3. Reduce the heat to low. Cover and simmer for about 15 minutes.

4. Season with required salt and black pepper.

SPLIT PEA SOUP

This is a filling soup full of protein from the peas. You may love to make it and freeze the extras for future rainy days! Garnish with chopped fresh cilantro leaves.

Serves: 2
Preparation Time: 15 minutes

Cooking Time: 53 minutes

Ingredients

- 1 tablespoon Water
- ½ small Yellow Onion, chopped
- 1 cup Green Split Peas
- 1 large Carrot, peeled and chopped
- 3 cups no-sodium Vegetable Broth
- ½ teaspoon Ground Cumin

- ¼ teaspoon Cayenne Pepper
- ¼ teaspoon Paprika
- Himalayan Salt, to taste
- Freshly Ground Black pepper, to taste

Directions

1. Heat the water in a large soup pan over a medium heat. Add the onion and sauté for 20 minutes, unless they become caramelized sooner.

2. Add all of the remaining ingredients and bring to a boil. Simmer on a low heat for 30 minutes, covered. Remove from heat and allow to slightly cool.

3. At the right temperature, place the soup in a blender and pulse until pureed. Return the soup to the pan. Stir in the lime juice and cook for 2 to 3 minutes.

CHILLED GREEN SOUP

This wonderfully delicious soup is ideal for a lunch time treat. The fresh green tomatoes are the key ingredient to making this a fantastic soup.

MAKES: 4 servings

PREPARATION TIME: 15 minutes (plus time to refrigerate)

Ingredients

- 2 pounds (450g) Ripe Green Tomatoes, chopped
- 1 large Cucumber peeled and chopped
- 1 Garlic Cloves, chopped
- 1 Jalapeño Pepper, seeded and chopped

- ¼ cup Cilantro Leaves, freshly chopped
- ¼ cup Basil Leaves, freshly chopped
- 1 tablespoon Fresh Lemon juice
- Pinch of Himalayan Pink Salt

Directions

1. Add the tomatoes to a blender and pulse until smooth. Strain the pureed tomatoes through a sieve into a large bowl.

2. Add the remaining ingredients to the blender and pulse until smooth. Slowly add the pureed tomatoes to the blender and pulse until smooth.

3. Transfer the soup into a large bowl and refrigerate for 2 to 4 hours before serving chilled.

CHILLED TANGY CUCUMBER SOUP

This is a wonderful and refreshing chilled cucumber soup. The use of fresh lime adds a delicate tangy taste while the fresh herbs provide a great taste.

MAKES: 4 servings

PREPARATION TIME: 15 minutes (plus time to refrigerate)

Ingredients

- 1 large Cucumber, peeled, seeded and chopped
- 1 small Scallion, chopped
- 2 tablespoons Mint Leaves, freshly chopped
- 2 tablespoons Parsley Leaves, freshly chopped
- ¼ teaspoon Lime Zest, freshly grated
- ½ tablespoon Fresh Lime juice
- 1¼ cups Filtered Water
- Pinch of Himalayan Pink Salt
- Pinch of Freshly Ground Black Pepper

Directions

1. Add all of the ingredients into a blender and pulse until smooth. Transfer the soup into a large bowl and cover and refrigerate for 4 to 6 hours.

2. Serve chilled.

BELL PEPPER & CASHEW SOUP

This nourishing soup is bursting with bright summer flavors. The cashews provide a nice creamy base to this bell pepper soup.

MAKES: 4 servings

PREPARATION TIME: 15 minutes

Ingredients

- ⅓ cup Green Bell Pepper, seeded and chopped
- ⅓ cup Red Bell Pepper, seeded and chopped
- ⅓ cup Raw Cashews, chopped
- ⅓ cup sodium-free Vegetable Broth
- ¼ teaspoon Fresh Lime juice

Directions

1. Add all of the ingredients into a blender and pulse until smooth.

2. Serve immediately.

FESTIVE AVOCADO SOUP

This cold and creamy avocado soup is velvety and smooth with a mild spicy kick. It is the perfect way to start a lavish summer dinner.

MAKES: 4 servings   **PREPARATION TIME:** 15 minutes

Ingredients

- 2 large Avocados, peeled, pitted and chopped
- 2 Scallions, chopped
- 2 Celery Stalks, chopped
- ½ cup Cilantro/Coriander Leaves, freshly chopped
- 1½ cups Filtered Water
- Pinch of Cayenne Pepper
- Pinch of Smoked Paprika
- Pinch of Himalayan Pink Salt
- Pinch of Freshly Ground Black Pepper

Directions

1. Add all of the ingredients into a blender and pulse until smooth.

2. Serve immediately.

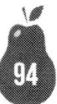

SPICY GREEN VEGETABLE SOUP

This recipe, having a combination of vegetables, spices and lemon is a fantastically healthy soup which is slightly tangy with a spicy flavor!

MAKES: 4 servings   **PREPARATION TIME:** 15 minutes

Ingredients

- 2 medium Zucchinis, peeled and chopped
- 6-8 Fresh Tomatoes, chopped
- 1 Green Bell Pepper, seeded and chopped
- 2-3 Celery Stalks, chopped
- 3 Scallions, chopped
- 1 tablespoon Basil Leaves, freshly chopped
- ½ teaspoon Lemon Zest, freshly grated
- 2 tablespoons Fresh Lemonjuice
- 1¼ cups Filtered Water
- ¼ teaspoon Ground Cumin
- Pinch of Cayenne Pepper
- Pinch of Freshly Ground Black Pepper

Directions

1. Add all of the ingredients into a blender and pulse until smooth.

2. Serve immediately.

BROCCOLI & AVOCADO SOUP

This is a healthy and tasty broccoli soup with a delightful spicy touch. The avocado also adds a wonderful creamy texture to this soup.

MAKES: 2 servings

PREPARATION TIME: 15 minutes

COOKING TIME: 40 minutes

Ingredients

- 3 cups (720ml) sodium-free Vegetable Broth
- 1 cup White Onion, chopped
- 2 Garlic Cloves, minced
- ¼ teaspoon Dried Thyme, crushed
- ¼ teaspoon Ground Cumin
- ¼ teaspoon Smoked Paprika
- Pinch of Cayenne Pepper
- 2 Heads Broccoli, cut into florets
- Pinch of Freshly Ground Black Pepper
- 1 Avocado, peeled, pitted and chopped

Directions

1. In a large soup pan, heat 2 tablespoons of the broth on a medium heat. Sauté the onion for 4 to 5 minutes before adding and sautéing the garlic, thyme and spices for 1 minute more. Stir in the broccoli and cook for 3 to 4 minutes. Add the remaining broth and bring to a boil on a high heat. Reduce the heat to medium-low and, whilst covered, simmer for 25 to 30 minutes.

2. Stir in the black pepper and remove from the heat and let the dish cool slightly. Transfer the broccoli mixture into a blender in batches. Add the avocado and pulse until smooth before serving immediately.

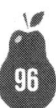

CURRIED PUMPKIN SOUP

This soup, which is wonderfully warming and comforting for the fall season, has a lovely subtle curry flavor.

MAKES: 4 servings
PREPARATION TIME: 15 minutes

COOKING TIME: 30 minutes

Ingredients

- 4 cups (960ml) sodium-free Vegetable Broth
- 1 medium Yellow Onion, chopped
- 2 Garlic Cloves, minced
- 2 teaspoons Ground Cumin
- ½ teaspoon Red Pepper Flakes, crushed
- 1 teaspoon Curry Powder

- 3 cups Pumpkin, peeled, seeded and chopped
- ¼ cups Almond Milk
- Pinch of Himalayan Pink Salt
- Freshly Ground Black Pepper, as required
- 1 tablespoon Fresh Lime juice

Directions

1. In a large soup pan, heat 2 tablespoons of the broth on a medium heat. Sauté the onion for 5 to 6 minutes. Add the garlic, cumin, red pepper flakes and curry powder and cook, stirring continuously, for 1 minute more.

2. Add the pumpkin and remaining broth and bring to a boil on a high heat. Reduce the heat to medium-low and simmer for 10 to 15 minutes. Stir in the almond milk and cook for 5 minutes. Season with salt and black pepper before removing from the heat and letting it cool slightly.

3. Transfer the mixture into a blender, in batches, and pulse until smooth. Return the soup to the pan and cook for 2 to 3 minutes, or until heated through. Transfer the soup into a serving bowl, stir in the lime juice and serve.

APPLE & CARROT SOUP

This is a winning combination of energeticand delicious ingredients! This thick and warming winter soup is extremely filling and tastes fantastic.

MAKES: 4 servings
PREPARATION TIME: 15 minutes

COOKING TIME: 36 minutes

Ingredients

- 4 cups(960ml) sodium-free Vegetable Broth
- 1 small White Onion, chopped
- 2 tablespoon Fresh Ginger, minced
- 1 Garlic Clove, minced
- 5 cups Carrots, peeled and chopped

- 2 small Apples, peeled, cored and chopped
- Pinch of Himalayan Pink Salt
- Freshly Ground Black Pepper, as required
- ¼ cup Parsley Leaves, freshly chopped

Directions

1. In a large soup pan, heat 2 tablespoons of the broth on a medium heat. Sauté the onion for 5 to 6 minutes before adding and sautéing the ginger and garlic for 1 minute more. Add 2 more tablespoons of the broth, stir in the carrots and apples and cook for 5 to 6 minutes. Add the remaining broth and bring to a boil on a high heat. Reduce the heat to medium-low and simmer for about 20 minutes. Remove the pan from the heat and let it cool slightly.

2. Transfer the mixture into a blender in batches and pulse until smooth. Return the soup to the pan and cook for a further 2 to 3 minutes, or until the soup is heated through. Stir in the salt, black pepper and parsley and serve.

POTATO & MUSHROOM SOUP

This is a wonderfully tasty and hearty soup filled with the great flavors of mushroom. This soup is really interesting and easy to prepare.

MAKES: 4 servings
PREPARATION TIME: 15 minutes

COOKING TIME: 35 minutes

Ingredients

- 4¼ cups (1litre) sodium-free Vegetable Broth
- 1 medium Yellow Onion, chopped
- 2-3 Garlic Cloves, minced
- ¼ teaspoon Dried Oregano, crushed
- ¼ teaspoon Dried Thyme, crushed
- ½ teaspoon Red Pepper Flakes, crushed

- 1 Potato, peeled and chopped
- 4 cups sliced, Fresh Baby Portobello Mushrooms
- ¼ cup Whole Wheat Flour
- Pinch of Himalayan Pink Salt
- Freshly Ground Black Pepper, as required
- 1 large Scallion, chopped

Directions

1. In a large soup pan, heat 2 tablespoons of the broth on a medium heat. Sauté the onion for 6 to 8 minutes before adding and sauté the garlic, herbsand red pepper flakes for 1 minute more. Add ¼ cup of broth, stir in the potato and mushrooms, and cook for 8 to 10 minutes. Stir in the wheat flour and cook, whilst stirring continuously, for about 1 minute more.

2. Add the remaining broth and bring to a boil on a high heat. Reduce the heat to medium-low and simmer for 10 to 15 minutes. Stir in the salt and black pepper, top with the scallions and serve.

SPICY CABBAGE SOUP

This simple and nourishing cabbage soup is delicious and will be a great hit for weight watchers!

MAKES: 4 servings
PREPARATION TIME: 15 minutes

COOKING TIME: 35 minutes

Ingredients

- 4 cups (960ml) sodium-free Vegetable Broth
- 1 small Yellow Onion, chopped
- 2 Garlic Cloves, minced
- 1teaspoon Ground Cumin
- ½ teaspoon Red Pepper Flakes, crushed
- 2 medium Carrots, finely chopped
- 1 cup Cabbage, shredded
- 1 cup Fresh Spinach, torn
- 1 cup Tomato Sauce
- Pinch of Himalayan Pink Salt
- Freshly Ground Black Pepper, as required
- 1 tablespoon Fresh Lime juice

Directions

1. In a large soup pan, heat 2 tablespoons of the broth on a medium heat. Sauté the onion for 4 to 5 minutes before adding and sautéing the garlic, cumin and red pepper flakes for 1 minute more. Add 2 tablespoons of the broth, stir in the carrot and cabbage and cook for a further 4 to 5 minutes.

2. Add the remaining broth and tomato sauce and bring to a boil on a high heat. Reduce the heat to medium-low and simmer for 15 to 20 minutes. Stir in the spinach and simmer for a further 3 to 4 minutes. Stir in salt, black pepper and lime juice and serve hot.

TOFU & MUSHROOM SOUP

This is a perfect healthy and delicious hit for a winter's cold night. The flavors of all the ingredients come together in a flash in this easy and super nutritious soup.

MAKES: 4 servings
PREPARATION TIME: 15 minutes

COOKING TIME: 10 minutes

Ingredients

- 3 cups (720ml) sodium-free Vegetable Broth
- 1 cup Tofu, pressed and cubed
- 2 cups Oyster Mushrooms, sliced
- ½ teaspoon Fresh Ginger, chopped
- 1 Jalapeño Pepper, seeded and chopped
- 4-5 Fresh Lime Leaves
- 1 medium Tomato, seeded and finely chopped
- 2 Scallions, chopped
- 1 teaspoon Low-Sodium Soy Sauce
- Pinch of Freshly Ground Black Pepper
- 2 tablespoons minced Cilantro Leaves
- 1 tablespoon Fresh Lime juice

Directions

1. In a large soup pan, add the broth and bring to a boil on a medium-high heat. Add the tofu, mushrooms, ginger, jalapeño and lime leaves. Reduce the heat to low and, whilst covered, simmer for about 5 minutes.

2. Stir in the remaining ingredients, except for the lime juice, and simmer for a further 2 to 3 minutes. Stir in the lime juice and serve hot.

CORN & POTATO SOUP

This is an easy to prepare soup recipe which is warm, healthy and satisfying. This wonderful soup is loaded with the subtle sweetness of corn.

MAKES: 4 servings
PREPARATION TIME: 15 minutes

COOKING TIME: 30 minutes

Ingredients

- 2¼ cups (520ml) sodium-free Vegetable Broth
- 1 medium Yellow Onion, chopped
- 2-3 Garlic Cloves, minced
- ½ teaspoon Red Pepper Flakes, crushed
- 1 small Russet Potato, peeled and chopped
- 3 Corn Ears, sliced
- 2 cups (480ml) unsweetened Almond Milk
- 2 tablespoons Nutritional Yeast
- Pinch of Himalayan Pink Salt
- Freshly Ground Black Pepper, as required
- 2 tablespoons minced Cilantro Leaves
- Pinch of Smoked Paprika

Directions

1. In a large soup pan, heat 2 tablespoons of the broth on a medium heat. Sauté the onion for 6 to 7 minutes before adding and sautéing the garlic and red pepper flakes for 1 minute more. Add 2 tablespoons of the broth, stir in the potato and cook for a further 4 to 5 minutes on a low heat. Stir in corn and cook for 1 to 2 minutes more.

2. Add the remaining broth and almond milk and bring to a boil on a medium-high heat. Reduce the heat to low and, whilst covered, simmer for about 5 minutes. Remove from the heat and let the dish cool slightly. Transfer half of the soup mixture into a blender and pulse until smooth. Return the soup into the pan and stir in the nutritional yeast. Cook for 10 minutes on a low heat. Stir in the salt and black pepper and remove from the heat.

3. Garnish with cilantro, sprinkle with paprika and serve hot.

CHICKPEA, QUINOA & VEGETABLE SOUP

This recipe makes a vibrant and comforting soup for the cold winter season. This soup is filled with the healthy proteins of quinoa, chickpeas and sweet potato, and has a lovely flavour from the spices.

MAKES: 4 servings

PREPARATION TIME: 15 minutes

COOKING TIME: 45 minutes

Ingredients

- 1½ cups (360ml) Filtered Water
- 1 cup Red Quinoa, rinsed and drained
- 6 cups Sodium free Vegetable Broth
- 1 medium Yellow Onion, chopped
- 2-3 Garlic Cloves, minced
- 1 Serrano Pepper, seeded and chopped
- 1teaspoon Ground Cumin
- ½ teaspoon Ground Cilantro
- ½ teaspoon Cayenne Pepper
- 2½ cups Sweet Potato, peeled and cubed into 1-inch size
- 1½ cups cooked Chickpeas
- 1 cup Fresh Spinach, torn
- Pinch of Himalayan Pink Salt
- Freshly Ground Black Pepper, as required
- ¼ cup Parsley Leaves, freshly chopped

Directions

1. In a pan, add the water and quinoa and bring to a boil on a high heat. Reduce the heat to medium and, whilst covered, simmer for about 17 minutes, or until the water has been completely absorbed. Remove the pan from the heat and fluff the quinoa with a fork before covering and setting aside.

2. In a large soup pan, heat 2 tablespoons of the broth on a medium heat. Sauté the onion for 6 to 8 minutes before adding and sautéing the garlic, Serrano pepper and spices for 1 minute more. Add 2 tablespoons of the broth, stir in the sweet potato and cook for 5 to 6 minutes. Add the remaining broth and bring to a boil on a medium-high heat before reducing the heat to medium and simmering for 18 to 20 minutes. Add the quinoa and the remaining ingredients, except for the parsley, and cook for a further 3 to 4 minutes.

3. Garnish with the parsley and serve.

HERBED BEANS SOUP

This festive soup, ideal for a winter holiday meal, tastes incredibly delicious and it warms the heart.

MAKES: 4 servings

PREPARATION TIME: 10 minutes

COOKING TIME: 35 minutes

Ingredients

- 4 cups (960ml) sodium-free Vegetable Broth
- 1 medium Onion, chopped
- 2 Celery Stalks, chopped
- 2 Carrots, peeled and chopped
- ½ teaspoon Fresh Ginger, minced
- 2-3 Garlic Cloves, minced
- 1 teaspoon Dried Thyme, crushed
- 1 teaspoon Dried Oregano, crushed
- 1½ cups cooked Red Kidney Beans
- 1½ cups cooked White Beans
- Pinch of Himalayan Pink Salt
- Freshly Ground Black Pepper, as required
- 1 tablespoon Fresh Lime juice
- ¼ cup Basil Leaves, freshly chopped

Directions

1. In a large soup pan, heat 3 tablespoons of the broth on a medium heat. Sauté the onion, celery and carrot for 4 to 5 minutes before adding and sautéing the garlic and herbs for 1 minute more. Add the remaining broth and beans and bring to a boil on a medium-high heat before reducing the heat to medium-low and simmering for 20 to 25 minutes.

2. Remove the pan from the heat and let it cool slightly. Transfer half of the soup mixture into a blender and pulse until smooth. Return the soup to the pan and cook for a further 3 to 4 minutes on a low heat. Stir in the salt, black pepper and lime juice before removing the pan from heat.

3. Garnish with basil and serve hot.

SPICY MIXED LENTIL SOUP

This protein packed and flavorful soup will be loved by the whole family, and it is guaranteed to keep you warm through the coldest weather.

MAKES: 4 servings
PREPARATION TIME: 15 minutes

COOKING TIME: 55 minutes

Ingredients

- 6 cups sodium-free Vegetable Broth
- 1 medium Onion, chopped
- 2 Celery Stalks, chopped
- 2-3 Garlic Cloves, minced
- 1teaspoon Ground Cumin
- ½ teaspoon Ground Cilantro
- ¼ teaspoon Ground Cinnamon
- ½ teaspoon Cayenne Pepper
- 1 cup Green Lentils, rinsed and drained
- ½ cup Black Lentils, rinsed and drained
- ½ cup Red Lentils, rinsed and drained
- Pinch of Himalayan Pink Salt
- Freshly Ground Black Pepper, as required
- ¼ cup Fresh Cilantro, chopped

Directions

1. In a large soup pan, heat 3 to 4 tablespoons of the broth on a medium heat. Sauté the onion and celery for 7 to 9 minutes before adding and sautéing the garlic and spices for 1 minute more. Add the remaining broth and all of the lentils and bring to a boil on a high heat. Reduce the heat to low and, whilst covered, simmer for 40 to 45 minutes.

2. Stir in the salt and black pepper. Garnish with the cilantro and serve hot.

PASTA & BEAN SOUP

This delicious soup is very easy to make and features navy beans, pasta and vegetables.

MAKES: 4 servings

PREPARATION TIME: 15 minutes
COOKING TIME: 45 minutes

Ingredients

- 4¼ cups (1 liter) sodium-free Vegetable Broth
- 2 cups Yellow Onion, chopped
- 2 Celery Stalks, chopped
- 1 medium Carrot, peeled and chopped
- 1 large Fresh Tomato, seeded and chopped

- 2 cups cooked Navy Beans
- 1 cup Whole Wheat Shell Pasta
- Pinch of Himalayan Pink Salt
- Freshly Ground Black Pepper, to taste
- 2 Scallions, chopped

Directions

1. In a large soup pan, heat 3 to 4 tablespoons of the broth on a medium heat. Sauté the onion, celery and carrot for 6 to 8 minutes. Add the tomato and cook for a further 1 to 2 minutes. Add the remaining broth and beans and bring to a boil on a high heat. Reduce the heat to medium-low and simmer for 20 to 25 minutes.

2. Add the pasta and cook for about 10 minutes. Stir in salt and black pepper, garnish with the scallion and serve hot.

DINNER RECIPES

HERBED GRAINS LOAF

This delicious and flavorful comfort food will even have your picky toddlers enjoying this grain loaf. The use of bulgur adds a lovely texture to this wonderful loaf.

MAKES: 4 servings
PREPARATION TIME: 15 minutes

COOKING TIME: 1 hour 15 minutes

Ingredients

- 1⅓ cups sodium-free Vegetable Broth
- ½ cup Brown Lentils
- 1 Bay Leaf
- 1 cup Boiled Water
- ¾ cup Bulgur
- ½ cup Tomato Sauce
- 1 cup Old-Fashioned Rolled Oats
- 2 tablespoons Ground Chia Seeds
- 2 tablespoons Nutritional Yeast

- 4 tablespoons Low-Sodium Soy Sauce
- 2 teaspoons Apple Cider Vinegar
- 2 tablespoons Sunflower Seed Butter
- 1 teaspoon Dried Basil, crushed
- ¼ teaspoon Dried Oregano, crushed
- ¼ teaspoon Dried Thyme, crushed
- Freshly Ground Black Pepper, as required

Directions

1. Preheat the oven to 375 degrees F and line a large loaf pan with parchment paper. In a pan, add the broth, lentils and bay leaf and bring to a boil on a high heat. Reduce the heat to medium-low and cook, covered, for 25 to 30 minutes. Add the boiling water and bulgur. Cook, covered, for 8 to 9 minutes. Remove from the heat and discard the bay leaf. Immediately stir in ¼ cup of tomato sauce and the remaining ingredients.

2. Transfer the lentil mixture into the prepared loaf pan and top with the remaining tomato sauce. Cover the pan with foil paper and bake for 25 to 28 minutes.

3. Remove the foil paper and bake for further 7 to 8 minutes.

LENTIL & RICE CASSEROLE

This simple and delicious casserole is quick to prepare and ideal for a family dinner.

MAKES: 4 servings
PREPARATION TIME: 10 minutes

COOKING TIME: 55 minutes

Ingredients

- 3 tablespoons Cashew Butter
- 2 tablespoons Filtered Water
- 1 small Onion, chopped
- 1 cup Mushrooms, chopped
- 1 Jalapeño Pepper, seeded and chopped
- 1 cup cooked Red Lentils
- 1 cup cooked Brown Rice
- 2 Whole Wheat Bread Slices, cubed
- ½ cup Cashew nuts, chopped
- 2 tablespoons Nutritional Yeast
- 2 teaspoons Mixed Dried Herbs (thyme, oregano, rosemary, sage), crushed
- ½ cup Rice Milk
- 1 cup sodium-free Vegetable Broth
- Freshly Ground Black Pepper, as required

Directions

1. Preheat the oven to 350 degrees F and grease a 9x8-inch casserole dish with 1 tablespoon of the cashew butter.

2. In a pan, heat the water on a medium heat. Sauté the onion and mushrooms for 8 to 9 minutes. Add the jalapeño pepper and sauté for about 1 minute more. Transfer the onion mixture into a large bowl. Add the remaining butter and ingredients and mix. Place the mixture into the prepared casserole dish.

3. Bake for about 45 minutes.

SPICY LENTILS & SWEET POTATO

This is a health boosting and very warming recipe for cold winter dinners. This dish is full of incredibly nourishing ingredients that really work well together.

MAKES: 4 servings
PREPARATION TIME: 15 minutes

COOKING TIME: 15 minutes

Ingredients

- 3 tablespoons Filtered Water
- 1 small Onion, chopped
- 2 Garlic Cloves, minced
- 1 teaspoon Fresh Ginger, minced
- ½ teaspoon Ground Cilantro
- ½ teaspoon Ground Cumin
- ½ teaspoon Red Pepper Flakes, crushed
- ½ teaspoon Red Chili Powder

- 1 cup Fresh Tomatoes, chopped finely
- ⅓ cup unsweetened Almond Milk
- 1 medium cooked Sweet Potato, peeled and cubed
- 1¾ cups Cooked Red Lentils
- 1 tablespoon Almond Butter
- 1 tablespoon Fresh Lime juice
- ¼ cup Parsley, freshly chopped

Directions

1. In a large pan, heat the water on a medium heat. Sauté the onion for 4 to 5 minutes before adding and sautéing the garlic, ginger and spices for 1 minute more. Add the tomatoes and, whilst stirring, cook for 3 to 4 minutes. Add the milk, potatoes and lentils and cook for a further 5 minutes.

2. Stir in the almond butter and lime juice, and remove the pan from the heat. Garnish with parsley and serve hot.

NUTTY BEANS & CELERY

This simple yet hearty vegan dish combines garbanzo beans with celery and spices to make a delicious meal for dinner.

MAKES: 4 servings
PREPARATION TIME: 15 minutes

COOKING TIME: 25 minutes

Ingredients

- 1½ cups sodium-free Vegetable Broth
- 1½ cups White Onion, chopped
- 3 Garlic Cloves, minced
- ¼ teaspoon Ground Cumin
- ¼ teaspoon Red Pepper Flakes, crushed
- 2 cups cooked Garbanzo Beans

- 3 cups Celery Root, peeled and chopped
- 1 tablespoon Fresh Lemon juice
- 2 tablespoons Almonds, chopped
- Freshly Ground Black Pepper, as required
- ¼ cup Fresh Cilantro, chopped

Directions

1. In a large pan, heat 3 tablespoons of the broth on a medium heat. Sauté the onion for 8 to 9 minutes before adding and sautéing the garlic and spices for 1 minute. Add the beans, celery and remaining broth. Bring the pan to a boil before reducing the heat and simmering for 15 minutes whilst covered.

2. Stir in the lemon juice, almonds and cilantro and remove from the heat. Season with black pepper and serve hot.

MIXED BEAN CHILI

This is anexcellentrecipe which combines the awesome flavors of mixed beans, bell peppers and spices. Even meat lovers will love to eat this delicious bean chili!

MAKES: 4 servings
PREPARATION TIME: 10 minutes

COOKING TIME: 30 minutes

Ingredients

- 1¼ cups sodium-free Vegetable Broth
- 1½ cups White Onion, chopped
- 3-4 Garlic Cloves, minced
- 2 teaspoons Ground Cumin
- 1 teaspoon Cayenne Pepper
- 2 teaspoons Red Chili Powder
- 1 small Green Bell Pepper, seeded and chopped
- 1 small Red Bell Pepper, seeded and chopped

- 1 small Yellow Bell Pepper, seeded and chopped
- 1 large Jalapeño Pepper, chopped
- 4 cups Fresh Tomatoes, finely chopped
- 1½ cups cooked Black Beans
- 1½ cups cooked White Beans
- 1½ cups cooked Red Kidney Beans
- ¼ cup Scallion, chopped

Directions

1. In a large pan, heat 2 tablespoons of the broth on a medium heat. Sauté the onion for 4 to 5 minutes before adding and sautéing the garlic and spices for 1 minute. Add 2 tablespoons of the broth, the bell peppers and the jalapeño pepper. Cook for 4 to 5 minutes whilst stirring occasionally. Add the tomatoes and, whilst stirring, cook for 3 to 4 minutes.

2. Add the remaining broth and the beans. Bring the dish to a boil before reducing the heat to low and simmering, covered, for 10 to 15 minutes. Top with the scallion and serve hot.

TOFU & BEAN FIESTA

This dish is a tasty and recipe for a hearty and filling dinner. It is packed with the protein punch of both beans and tofu.

MAKES: 4 servings
PREPARATION TIME: 10 minutes

COOKING TIME: 30 minutes

Ingredients

- 1 cup Filtered Water
- 1½ cups White Onion, chopped
- 2 Garlic Cloves, minced
- 1 Green Chili, chopped
- 1 teaspoon Ground Cumin
- ½ teaspoon Red Chili Powder
- 1 Stalk Celery, chopped
- 1 small Green Bell Pepper, seeded and chopped

- 1 Carrot, peeled and chopped
- 12-ounces Firm Tofu, pressed and chopped
- 1¾ cups Tomatoes, chopped
- 1½ cups cooked Red Kidney Beans
- 3 tablespoons Fresh Cilantro, chopped

Directions

1. In a large pan, heat 2 tablespoons of the water on a medium heat. Sauté the onion for 4 to 5 minutes before adding and sautéing the garlic, green chili and spices for 1 minute. Add the vegetables and sauté for 3 to 4 minutes. Add 2 tablespoons of water and the tofu and cook, stirring, for 8 to 10 minutes.

2. Add the remaining water, tomatoes and beans. Bring the dish to a boil before reducing the heat to low and simmering, covered, for about 10 minutes. Top with the cilantro and serve hot.

SPICY BEAN STEW

This stew is a great hit for holiday dinners. It has a great tasting combination of beans and corn with the unique flavor of the spices.

MAKES: 4 servings
PREPARATION TIME: 20 minutes

COOKING TIME: 1 hour 40 minutes

Ingredients

- 6 cups sodium-free Vegetable Broth
- 1 cup White Onion, chopped
- ½ cup Celery, chopped
- 3-4 Garlic Cloves, minced
- 1 Jalapeño Pepper, chopped
- 1 teaspoon Fresh Ginger, minced
- ½ teaspoon Ground Cilantro
- ½ teaspoon Ground Cumin
- ½ teaspoon Red Pepper Flakes, crushed
- ½ teaspoon Red Chili Powder
- 1 Red Bell Pepper, seeded and chopped
- 1 Green Bell Pepper, seeded and chopped
- ½ cup Carrot, peeled and chopped
- 2 cups Fresh Corn Kernels
- 1 cup Dried Red Kidney Beans, soaked overnight and drained
- ¼ cup Basil Leaves, freshly chopped

Directions

1. In a large pan, heat 2 tablespoons of the broth on a medium heat. Sauté the onion for 4 to 5 minutes before adding and sautéing the garlic, jalapeño pepper and spices for 1 minute. Add 2 tablespoons of the broth and the vegetables, and sauté for a further 3 to 4 minutes.

2. Add the remaining broth, corn and beans, and bring to a boil. Reduce the heat to low and simmer, covered, for 1 to 1½ hours. Top with the basil and serve hot.

SPICY VEGETABLE STEW

This is a great recipe for a perfect warming dinner meal. This easy and flavorful mixed vegetable stew gets its delicious kick from the combination of all the spices that are used.

MAKES: 4 servings
PREPARATION TIME: 20 minutes

COOKING TIME: 40 minutes

Ingredients

- 4¼ cups sodium-free Vegetable Broth
- 1½ cups White Onion, chopped
- 2 Garlic Cloves, minced
- ½ teaspoon Fresh Ginger, minced
- ½ teaspoon Ground Cilantro
- ½ teaspoon Ground Cumin
- ⅛ teaspoon Ground Cinnamon
- Pinch of Ground Cloves
- ½ teaspoon Red Chili Powder
- ½ teaspoon Smoked Paprika
- 2 cups Fresh Tomatoes, finely chopped
- 2 cups Potatoes, peeled and chopped
- 2 cups carrots, peeled and chopped
- 1 small peeled, seeded and chopped Butternut Squash
- 2 cups Green Bell Pepper, seeded and chopped
- Pinch of Himalayan Pink Salt
- 1 tablespoon Fresh Lemon juice
- ¼ cup Cilantro, freshly chopped

Directions

1. In a large pan, heat 2 tablespoons of the broth on a medium heat. Sauté the onion for 4 to 5 minutes before adding and sautéing the garlic and spices for 1 additional minute. Add the tomatoes and cook, stirring, for 3 to 4 minutes. Add 2 more tablespoons of the broth and the vegetables and cook, stirring occasionally, for 4 to 5 minutes.

2. Add the remaining broth and bring the pan to a boil before reducing the heat to medium-low and simmering, covered, for 20 to 25 minutes.

3. Stir in salt, lemon juice and cilantro. Remove the dish from the heat and serve hot.

CURRIED SQUASH & KALE

This is an absolutely delicious vegetable curry. The butternut squash and kale provide a lovely combination with the curry powder and almond milk.

MAKES: 4 servings
PREPARATION TIME: 15 minutes

COOKING TIME: 35 minutes

Ingredients

- 2 tablespoons Sodium free Vegetable Broth
- 1½ cups White Onion, chopped
- 3-4 Garlic Cloves, minced
- 2 tablespoons Curry Powder
- ½ teaspoon Ground Cumin
- 2 cups Filtered Water

- 4 cups peeled, seeded and cubed Butternut Squash
- 1 cup unsweetened Almond Milk
- 3 cups Fresh Kale, trimmed and chopped
- Freshly Ground Black Pepper, as required

Directions

1. In a large pan, heat the broth on a medium heat. Sauté the onion for 4 to 5 minutes before adding and sautéing the garlic, curry powder and cumin for 1 minute more. Add the water and squash and bring the pan to a boil before reducing the heat to low and simmering, covered, for 20 to 25 minutes.

2. Add the almond milk and return to a boil on a medium heat. Stir in the kale and cook for 3 to 4 minutes. Season with black pepper and serve hot.

ROASTED MIXED VEGETABLES

These roasted vegetables serve up a healthy and tasty vegetable dinner. They are infused with the flavors of almond butter, lemon juice and rosemary.

MAKES: 4 servings
PREPARATION TIME: 20 minutes

COOKING TIME: 40 minutes

Ingredients

- 1¼ cups Portobello Mushrooms, sliced
- 2 large Zucchinis, halved lengthwise and sliced
- 2 medium Carrots, peeled and chopped
- 1 medium Head Broccoli , cut into florets
- 1 medium Head Cauliflower, cut into florets
- 1 large Red Bell Pepper, seeded and sliced
- 1 cup Grape Tomatoes, halved
- ¼ cup Almond Butter
- 1 teaspoon Dried Rosemary, crushed
- 1 tablespoon Fresh Lemon juice
- Pinch Himalayan Pink Salt
- ½ teaspoon Red Pepper Flakes, crushed
- Freshly Ground Black Pepper, as required

Directions

1. Preheat the oven to 425 degrees F and line 2 roasting pans with foil paper.

2. In a large bowl, mix together all of the ingredients. Transfer the vegetable mixture into the prepared roasting pans. Roast for 35 to 40 minutes, tossing the vegetables every 15 minutes.

MIXED VEGETABLE CASSEROLE

This is a fantastic recipe for an extremely comforting and delicious casserole. This classic dish will be a great hit for special dinner parties.

MAKES: 4 servings
PREPARATION TIME: 20 minutes

COOKING TIME: 1 hour 5 minutes

Ingredients

For Topping:
- 3 pounds Red Potatoes, peeled and chopped
- 1 small Garlic Clove, minced
- 1½ cups Almond Milk
- 2 tablespoons Almond Butter
- Pinch Himalayan Pink Salt
- Freshly Ground Black Pepper, as required
- 1 teaspoon Dried Oregano, crushed
- ½ teaspoon Red Pepper Flakes, crushed

For Filling:
- 2 tablespoons Almond Butter

- 1 cup White Onion, chopped
- 4 Celery Stalks, chopped
- 2-3 Garlic Cloves, minced
- 1½ teaspoons Mixed Dried Herbs (thyme, oregano, rosemary, basil), crushed
- 1 Turnip, peeled and chopped
- 1 Parsnip, peeled and chopped
- 3-4 medium Carrots, peeled and chopped
- 1¼ cups Sodium free Vegetable Broth
- 3 tablespoons Whole Wheat Flour
- Pinch Himalayan Pink Salt
- Freshly Ground Black Pepper, as required

Directions

1. Preheat the oven to 425 degrees F and grease a large casserole dish with some almond butter. In a pan of boiling water, add the potatoes and cook on low heat for 25 to 30 minutes. Drain well and transfer into a large bowl. With a fork mash the potatoes before mixing in the garlic, almond milk, butter, salt and black pepper and setting aside.

2. Meanwhile, for the filling, in a large skillet melt the butter on a medium heat. Add the onion and celery and sauté for 3 to 4 minutes. Add garlic and herbs and sauté for 1 minute more. Add the vegetables and cook for 10 to 15 minutes. In a bowl, mix together the broth, flour and seasoning. Add the broth mixture into the skillet and cook, stirring occasionally, for 5 to 10 minutes.

3. Transfer the vegetable mixture into the prepared casserole dish and place the potato mixture over the vegetables. Sprinkle with crushed oregano and red pepper flakes and bake for about 35 minutes, or until the top has become golden brown.

PASTA WITH BROCCOLI

This is a super quick, satisfying and delicious pasta dish for family and friends. The flavors of the pasta, broccoli rabe and fresh thyme pair wonderfully with the chickpeas.

MAKES: 2 servings
PREPARATION TIME: 10 minutes

COOKING TIME: 15 minutes

Ingredients

- 1½ cups Whole Wheat Pasta
- ½ bunch Broccoli Rabe, trimmed and cut into bite size pieces
- ¾ cup sodium-free Vegetable Broth
- 3-4 Garlic Cloves, minced
- ½ teaspoon Thyme, freshly chopped

- 2 teaspoons Whole Wheat Flour
- 1 cup cooked White Beans
- 2 teaspoons Fresh Lemon juice
- Pinch Himalayan Pink Salt
- Freshly Ground Black Pepper, as required

Directions

1. In a large pan of boiling water, add the pasta and cook for 5 to 6 minutes. Add the broccoli rabe and cook for a further 3 minutes. Drain well and Set aside.

2. In a large skillet, heat 1 tablespoon of the broth on a medium heat. Sauté the garlic and thyme for about 1 minute. Stir in the remaining broth and flour. Bring to a boil whilst stirring continuously. Reduce the heat to medium-low and cook for 2 minutes.

3. Stir in the pasta mixture and remaining ingredients. Cook, stirring, for 2 to 3 minutes more before serving.

MILLET WITH MUSHROOM & SPINACH

This is an easy yet fabulous dish for the colder winter months. This recipe is full of delicious nutrient-rich ingredients.

MAKES: 2 servings
PREPARATION TIME: 10 minutes

COOKING TIME: 25 minutes

Ingredients

- 1½ cups Sodium free Vegetable Broth
- 2 cups Yellow Onion, chopped
- 2 small Garlic Cloves, minced
- 1 Jalapeño Pepper, seeded and chopped
- 1½ tablespoons Fresh Thyme, chopped
- 4 cups Shiitake Mushrooms, sliced

- 1½ tablespoons Low-Sodium Soy Sauce
- 2 tablespoons Nutritional Yeast
- ½ tablespoon Corn Starch
- 1 cup Fresh Spinach, chopped
- Freshly Ground Black Pepper, as required
- 2 cups cooked Millet

Directions

1. In a large skillet, heat 2 tablespoons of broth on a medium heat. Sauté the onion for 4 to 5 minutes before adding and sautéing the garlic, jalapeño and thyme for 1 minute more. Add 2 tablespoons of the broth and the mushrooms and sauté for a further 10 minutes. Sir in the soy sauce and nutritional yeast and cook for 2 to 3 minutes.

2. Meanwhile, in a bowl mix together the corn starch and remaining broth. Add the broth mixture and spinach into the skillet with the mushrooms and cook for 5 to 6 minutes, or until the gravy is thickened to your liking.

3. Place the millet on a serving plate, top with the mushroom and spinach gravy and serve.

CURRIED TOFU & BEANS

An incredibly delicious and filling meal, this hearty vegetarian dish is flavored with a wonderful spice combination that will leave your kitchen smelling incredible! Garnish with chopped cilantro.

Serves: 2
Prep Time: 10 minutes

Cooking Time: 26 minutes

Ingredients

- 2 tablespoons Water
- 1 small Onion, chopped
- 1 teaspoon Fresh Ginger, minced
- 2 Garlic Cloves, minced
- Pinch of Cayenne Pepper
- ½ teaspoon Ground Cumin
- 2 teaspoons Curry Powder
- ½ cup no-sodium Vegetable Broth
- 8-ounces Firm Tofu, pressed and cubed
- 1 cup Tomato, chopped finely
- ½ Head Cauliflower, cut into bite size pieces
- 1 cup Cooked Garbanzo Beans
- Himalayan Salt, to taste
- 1 tablespoon Fresh Lime juice

Directions

1. In a large pan, heat the water on a medium heat. Add the onion and sauté for 4 to 5 minutes. Add the ginger, garlic, cayenne pepper, cumin and curry powder, and sauté for 1 minute.

2. Add the broth, tofu, tomato and cauliflower, and bring to the boil. Cover the pan and simmer for 10 minutes on a low heat.

3. Stir in the beans and salt, and simmer for 10 minutes.

4. Stir in the lime juice and serve hot.

DESSERT RECIPES

BROWN RICE PUDDING

This is an excellent dessert for promoting good health. The combination of ingredients in this pudding makes a slightly nutty and delicious dessert.

MAKES: 4 servings

PREPARATION TIME: 10 minutes (plus time to chill)

COOKING TIME: 45 minute

Ingredients

- 2 cups Filtered Water
- 1 cup Brown Rice, rinsed
- ⅓ cup Pure Maple Syrup
- 1¼ cups unsweetened Almond Milk
- ⅓ cup Golden Raisins
- ½ teaspoon Ground Cinnamon

- Pinch of Ground Nutmeg
- Pinch of Ground Ginger
- Pinch of Ground Cloves
- Pinch of Pink Himalayan Salt
- 2 tablespoons Almonds, toasted and chopped

Directions

1. In a pan, add the water and bring to a boil on a medium-high heat. Add the rice and reduce the heat to low and simmer, covered, for about 35 minutes. Stir in the remaining ingredients and cook for a further 5 to 10 minutes, or until all of the water has gone.

2. Transfer the rice pudding into a serving bowl. Refrigerate to chill completely before topping with the almonds and serving.

BANANA ICE CREAM CAKE

This is an easy and delicious dessert for that sweet tooth. Kids will love to eat this simple homemade ice cream cake! This a perfect treat on a special occasion or holiday.

MAKES: 4 servings

PREPARATION TIME: 15 minutes (plus time to chill)

Ingredients

- 1 cup Raw Cashew Nuts
- 1 cup Medjool Dates, pitted and chopped

- 2 Bananas, peeled and sliced

Directions

1. Line a small baking tin with parchment paper.

2. In a food processor, add the cashew nuts and pulse until finely chopped. Add the dates and bananas and pulse until smooth.

3. Transfer the mixture into the prepared baking tin and freeze to chill the cake. Cut into your desired size slices before serving.

KIWI SORBET

Sweet and tart kiwis gives this refreshing dessert its brilliant green color and smooth texture. This is a fantastic sorbet to end any meal.

MAKES: 4 servings

PREPARATION TIME: 10 minutes (plus time to chill)

Ingredients

- 8 Kiwis, peeled and chopped
- 3 tablespoons Pure Maple Syrup
- 1½ tablespoons Fresh Lime or Lemon juice

Directions

1. Place all of the ingredients into a blender and pulse until smooth. Transfer the mixture into a bowl, cover and freeze to chill for at least 1 hour.

2. Transfer the solution into an ice cream maker and process according to the manufacturer's directions. Transfer into an air tight container, cover and freeze to chill completely before serving.

RASPBERRY CHIA PARFAIT

This is a delicious and healthy combination of chia seeds and raspberries with cinnamon and vanilla. This recipe makes a beautiful, fancy and great tasting parfait.

MAKES: 2 servings

PREPARATION TIME: 10 minutes (plus time to chill)

Ingredients

- 2 cups (480ml) Unsweetened Almond Milk
- 2 tablespoons Pure Maple Syrup
- ⅛ teaspoon Vanilla Extract
- ¼ teaspoon Ground Cinnamon
- Pinch of Pink Himalayan Salt
- ¾ cup Fresh Raspberries
- ⅓ cup Chia Seeds
- 1 tablespoon Walnuts, toasted and chopped

Directions

1. In a blender, add the almond milk, maple syrup, vanilla, cinnamon and salt and pulse until mixed. Add the chia seeds and briefly pulse to mix. Add ½ cup of raspberries and pulse until blended.

2. Transfer the mixture into a serving bowl. Cover and refrigerate to chill for at least 5 to 6 hours, stirring occasionally. Top with the remaining raspberries and walnuts before serving.

TOFU CUSTARD

This simple, quick, subtle and yummy custard will satisfy anyone with a sweet tooth.

MAKES: 2 servings

PREPARATION TIME: 10 minutes (plus time to chill)

Ingredients

- 12-ounces Silken Tofu, pressed
- 3 tablespoons organic Almond Butter
- 1 teaspoon Vanilla Extract
- ⅛ teaspoon Ground Cinnamon
- Pinch of Pink Himalayan Salt
- ⅓ cup Pure Maple Syrup
- Additional Ground Cinnamon, for sprinkling

Directions

1. Place all of the ingredients into a blender and pulse until smooth. Transfer the mixture into a serving bowl. Cover and refrigerate to chill for at least 5 to 6 hours whilst stirring occasionally.

2. Sprinkle with cinnamon and serve.

CITRUS QUINOA PUDDING

This healthy dessert is packed with proteins from the quinoa and plump raisins. The citrus juices in this pudding add a refreshingly tangy twist.

MAKES: 4 servings
PREPARATION TIME: 15 minutes

COOKING TIME: 30 minute

Ingredients

- 2 cups Filtered Water
- 1 cup Red Quinoa, rinsed and drained
- 1 cup Golden Raisins
- 2 cups fresh unsweetened Apple Juice
- 1 tablespoon Fresh Lemon juice

- 1 tablespoon Fresh Lime juice
- 2 teaspoons Vanilla Extract
- Pinch of Pink Himalayan Salt
- 2 tablespoons Pistachios, roughly chopped
- 1 teaspoon Orange Zest, freshly grated

Directions

1. In a pan, add the water and quinoa and bring to a boil on a high heat. Reduce the heat, cover and simmer for about 15 minutes. Stir in the remaining ingredients, except for the pistachios and orange zest. Cover and simmer for a further 15 minutes.

2. Transfer into serving bowls. Top with the pistachios and orange zest and serve warm.

BAKED PUMPKIN BREAD PUDDING

This pudding is a delicious blend of bread, pumpkin puree and warm spices. It is easy to make and tastes fantastic.

MAKES: 4 servings
PREPARATION TIME: 15 minutes

COOKING TIME: 30 minute

Ingredients

- ½ cup unsweetened Almond Milk, warmed
- ½ teaspoon Apple Cider Vinegar
- 2 tablespoons Golden Flax Meal

For Bread Pudding:
- 1 cup Homemade Pumpkin Puree
- ⅓ cup Almond Milk
- ¼ cup Pure Maple Syrup

- 1 teaspoon Ground Cinnamon
- ½ teaspoon Ground Ginger
- ½ teaspoon Ground Nutmeg
- ¼ teaspoon Ground Cloves
- Pinch of Pink Himalayan Salt
- 5 cups cubed, stale Whole Wheat Bread Slices
- ½ cup Almond Butter

Directions

1. Preheat the oven to 350 degrees F. In a small bowl, mix together the warm almond milk, vinegar and flax meal. Set aside for at least 5 minutes.

2. In another large bowl, beat together the pumpkin puree, milk, maple syrup and spices. Stir in the flax meal mixture. Place the bread cubes into a third bowl, add the butter and thoroughly coat the cubes. Add the pumpkin mixture and mix well before transferring the mixture into a baking dish and baking for 25 to 30 minutes.

VANILLA MUG CAKE

This is a delicious mug cake which has a definite moist deliciousness, looks great and will be loved by all vanilla lovers!

MAKES: 2 servings
PREPARATION TIME: 10 minutes

COOKING TIME: 1 minute

Ingredients

- ¼ cup Whole Wheat Flour
- ½ teaspoon Baking Powder
- ½ teaspoon Ground Cinnamon
- Pinch of Pink Himalayan Salt
- ¼ cup unsweetened Almond Milk

- 2 tablespoons organic Almond Butter
- 2 tablespoons Pure Maple Syrup
- ½ teaspoon Vanilla Extract

Directions

1. In a bowl, mix together the baking powder, flour, cinnamon and salt. In another bowl, add the remaining ingredients and beat until well combined. Mix the milk mixture into the flour mixture.

2. Transfer the mixture into 2 microwave safe mugs and microwave on high for about 1 minute.

AVOCADO CHEESECAKE

This recipe makes a wonderfully yummy and nutrient filled cheesecake. It uses the avocado, an amazingly healthy and creamy fruit, to create a wonderfully delicious dessert.

MAKES: 2 servings

PREPARATION TIME: 10 minutes (plus time to freeze)

Ingredients

For Crust:
- ⅓ cup Dates, pitted and chopped
- ½ cup Walnuts, soaked and drained
- 1 teaspoon Filtered Water

For Filling:
- 1 large Avocado, peeled, pitted and chopped
- ½ teaspoon fresh Lemon Zest

- ¼ cup organic Almond Butter
- ¼ cup Pure Maple Syrup
- ½ tablespoon Fresh Lemon juice

For Topping:
- 1½ cups Frozen Raspberries
- 1 tablespoon Pure Maple Syrup
- ¼ tablespoon Fresh Lemon juice

Directions

1. Grease a small pie dish with some almond butter. For the crust, add all of the crust ingredients into a food processor and pulse until smooth. Transfer the mixture into the prepared pie dish, pressing downwards gently. In a blender, add all of the filling ingredients and pulse until smooth and creamy. Evenly place the filling mixture over the crust and freeze for at least 4 to 6 hours, or until the filling has set.

2. Add all of the topping ingredients into a blender and pulse until smooth. Spread the topping over the filling mixture and freeze until set.

LEMONY APPLE BITES

This easy to prepare apple dessert is really light and sweet without using any sweetener. This flavorful and nutritional recipe will be a great addition to any fall desserts.

MAKES: 4 servings   **PREPARATION TIME:** 15 minutes

Ingredients

For Apples:
- 3 Apples, cored and cubed
- 1 tablespoon Fresh Lemon juice

For Sauce:
- 2 Apples, cored and chopped
- 6 Medjool Dates, pitted and chopped

- 2 tablespoons Fresh Lemon juice
- ¼ teaspoon Ground Nutmeg
- ¼ teaspoon Ground Cinnamon

For Topping:
- 2 large Dates, pitted and chopped
- ½ cup Pecans, chopped
- 1 teaspoon fresh Lemon Zest

Directions

1. In a large bowl, add the cubed apples and drizzle with the lemon juice before setting aside. In a food processor, add all of the sauce ingredients and pulse until smooth. Pour the sauce over the cubed apples and toss to coat well. Transfer the mixture into serving bowls.

2. For the topping, add the dates and pecans into a food processor and pulse until smooth. Top the Apple mixture with the pecan mixture. Sprinkle with lemon zest and serve.

BERRY CRISP

This recipe is an ideal and great tasting way to use seasonal fresh berries. This delicious crisp has a juicy filling of mixed fresh berries.

MAKES: 4 servings
PREPARATION TIME: 15 minutes

COOKING TIME: 30 minutes

Ingredients

For Filling:
- 1 cup Fresh Strawberries, hulled and sliced
- 1 cup Fresh Raspberries
- 1 cup Fresh Blueberries
- 1 cup Fresh Blackberries
- 6 Medjool Dates, pitted and finely chopped
- ¾ cup Filtered Water
- ½ teaspoon Vanilla Extract

- ½ teaspoon Ground Nutmeg
- ½ teaspoon Ground Cinnamon

For Topping:
- 1¼ cups Rolled Oats
- ¼ cup Pecans, roughly chopped
- 3 Medjool Dates, pitted and finely chopped
- ½ teaspoon Ground Cinnamon
- 2 tablespoons Filtered Water

Directions

1. Preheat the oven to 375 degrees F and lightly grease a baking dish with the almond butter.

2. In a large bowl, add all of the filling ingredients and toss to combine well. Transfer the mixture into the prepared baking dish.

3. In a food processor, add all of the topping ingredients and pulse until well combined. Evenly spread the topping mixture over the filling mixture, pressing down slightly. Bake for about 30 minutes, or until the top has become a golden brown color.

LAYERED FRUIT & NUT TREAT

This delicious dessert is a healthy combination of nuts and fresh fruit.

MAKES: 2 servings
PREPARATION TIME: 15 minutes

COOKING TIME: 1 minute 15 seconds

Ingredients

For Nutty Layer
- 2 Dates, pitted and chopped
- ¼ cup Cashew nuts
- ¼ cup Almonds, chopped
- 1 tablespoon Almond Butter
- Pinch of Ground Nutmeg
- ½ teaspoon Ground Cinnamon
- ⅛ teaspoon Vanilla Extract
- 2 tablespoons Filtered Water

For Fruity Layer
- ½ Apple, peeled, cored and sliced thinly
- ½ Pear, peeled, cored and sliced thinly
- 3 tablespoons Fresh Lemon juice
- 1 teaspoon Ground Cinnamon

Directions

1. In a food processor, add the nutty layer ingredients and pulse until smooth. Transfer the mixture into 2 bowls. For the fruity layer, add the fruit slices and lemon juice into a microwave safe bowl and microwave on high for about 45 seconds before stirring in the cinnamon.

2. Place half of the nut mixture into two microwave safe bowls. Place the fruit mixture over nut mixture and top with the remaining nut mixture. Microwave on high for 30 seconds before serving warm.

EASY CONVERSION CHART

This cookbook is for everyone! Hence, this measurement conversion chart is included to enhance the overall user experience of this recipe book. Particularly, readers who are living in the UK will find this conversion chart to be quite helpful for easily converting any of these recipes.

FOR LIQUID INGREDIENTS
1 teaspoon (tsp) = 6 milliliters (ml)
1 tablespoon (tbsp) = 15 milliliters (ml)
1/8 cup = 30 milliliters (ml)
¼ cup = 60 milliliters (ml)
½ cup = 120 milliliters (ml)
1 cup = 240 milliliters (ml)

FOR DRY OR SOLID INGREDIENTS
1 teaspoon (tsp) = 5 grams (g)
1 tablespoon (tbsp) = 15 grams (g)
1 ounce (oz) = 28 grams (g)
1 cup flour = 150 grams (g)
1 cup sugar = 175 grams (g)

1 cup spiralized fruit or vegetable = 175 grams (g)
1 small spiralized courgette, fruit or other vegetable = 120 -150 grams (g)
1 medium spiralized courgette, fruit or vegetable = 195 -225 grams (g)
1 large spiralized courgette, fruit or vegetable = 250 -315 grams (g)
 1 cup nuts or seeds = 200 grams (g)
1/8 cup butter = 30 grams (g)
¼ cup butter = 55 grams (g)
1/3 cup butter = 75 grams (g)
½ cup butter = 115 grams (g)
2/3 cup butter = 150 grams (g)
¾ cup butter = 170 grams (g)
1 cup butter = 225 grams (g)

OVEN TEMPERATURES
275° Fahrenheit (F) = 140° Celsius (C) or Gas Mark 1
300° Fahrenheit (F) = 150° Celsius (C) or Gas Mark 2
325° Fahrenheit (F) = 165° Celsius (C) or Gas Mark 3
350° Fahrenheit (F) = 180° Celsius (C) or Gas Mark 4
375° Fahrenheit (F) = 190° Celsius (C) or Gas Mark 5
400° Fahrenheit (F) = 200° Celsius (C) or Gas Mark 6
425° Fahrenheit (F) = 220° Celsius (C) or Gas Mark 7
450° Fahrenheit (F) = 230° Celsius (C) or Gas Mark 8

SAVING HEARTS—SAVING LIVES!

Remember that there are no magic bullets for a good heart or for good health in general. If you really want to enjoy good health, you will have to change your lifestyle. You will have to choose to win. There is no way of getting around that. Preventing and reversing heart disease requires permanent change to your everyday lifestyle. Even if you drift a bit from this diet on special occasions or holidays that won't hurt. What is more important is your regular eating habit. That's where the real results will come from.

By now, we can agree that how we eat seriously affects our heart. Heart disease is a dietary disease and should be taken very seriously. Therefore, let's stop shoving all the junk food into our system and start flooding our system with live enzymes from real food. With this cookbook of over 100 heart healthy recipes, you are now equipped with an effective weapon to combat mankind's worst killer. In reality, we live in a very seductive world. But always remember that despite all the food seduction, you have the power of choice. You are largely determining how long you want to live and which disease you want to have by the choices that you make. It is highly unlikely that you will get a heart attack if you start eating properly. Amazing isn't it?

I am thrilled that you have chosen to use my book on your quest to better heart health. Thank you! I would be delighted if you would share your experience with other readers. You can eat your way out of heart disease!

From my kitchen to yours,
Elizabeth Holm

Printed in Great Britain
by Amazon